HAND
REFLEXOLOGY

Denise Whichello Brown

S

Acknowledgements

My thanks to the publishers, Hodder & Stoughton, for allowing me to write yet another book. My love and thanks to my dear husband, Garry, and my two beloved children, Chloe and Thomas. Thanks also to all my patients and students who have taught me so much over the years. Finally I thank all the higher energies of the cosmos that guide me in my work, especially Sai Baba, and my angels and archangels, Melchizedek and Kwan Yin. I feel truly blessed to be graced by their presence and unconditional love so that I may radiate fully the love and light of my being.

For UK order queries: please contact Bookpoint Ltd, 130 Milton Park, Abingdon, Oxon OX14 4SB. Telephone: (44) 01235 827720. Fax: (44) 01235 400454. Lines are open from 9.00–18.00, Monday to Saturday, with a 24-hour message answering service. Email address: orders@bookpoint.co.uk

For U.S.A. order queries: please contact McGraw-Hill Customer Services, P.O. Box 545, Blacklick, OH 43004-0545, U.S.A. Telephone: 1-800-722-4726. Fax: 1-614-755-5645.

For Canada order queries: please contact McGraw-Hill Ryerson Ltd., 300 Water St, Whitby, Ontario L1N 9B6, Canada. Telephone: 905 430 5000. Fax: 905 430 5020.

Long renowned as the authoritative source for self-guided learning – with more than 30 million copies sold worldwide – the *Teach Yourself* series includes over 300 titles in the fields of languages, crafts, hobbies, business and education.

British Library Cataloguing in Publication Data
A catalogue record for this title is available from The British Library.

Library of Congress Catalog Card Number: On file

First published in UK 2002 by Hodder Headline Plc, 338 Euston Road, London, NW1 3BH.

First published in US 2002 by Contemporary Books, A Division of The McGraw-Hill Companies, 4255 West Touhy Avenue, Lincolnwood (Chicago), Illinois 60712–1975 U.S.A.

The 'Teach Yourself' name and logo are registered trade marks of Hodder & Stoughton Ltd.

Typeset by Transet Limited, Coventry, England.
Printed in Great Britain for Hodder & Stoughton Educational, a division of Hodder Headline Plc, 338 Euston Road, London NW1 3BH by Cox & Wyman Ltd, Reading, Berkshire.

Impression number   10 9 8 7 6 5 4 3 2 1
Year   2007 2006 2005 2004 2003 2002

CONTENTS

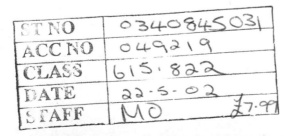

INTRODUCTION

Teach Yourself Hand Reflexology is a simple, straightforward, practical guide to this ancient and increasingly popular healing art.

It is invaluable for the layperson as a means of self-help. The techniques described in this book will enable you to safely eliminate most common aliments, whether physical or emotional. No special equipment is required and you can treat yourself as well as your friends and family easily and effectively. You will be amazed at the results that can be achieved, regardless of your inexperience. Hand reflexology will quickly become part of your daily routine, as it has mine!

This easy-to-follow guide will also appeal to budding reflexologists who are embarking upon professional training as well as those who are fully qualified. Many books have been written on foot reflexology but very few on hand reflexology. This book is a must for any reflexologist's library and may open your eyes to new ways of treating your patients. Hand reflexology is just as effective as foot reflexology and there are some instances when it may be impossible to work on the feet. In my own practice I use a combination of hand and foot reflexology with outstanding results. If the clients are instructed to work on their own hands between treatments, this reinforces the treatment you are giving. The healing forces are speeded up dramatically and patients recover remarkably quickly. They also develop a sense of responsibility towards their own health which is important if optimum health is to be maintained.

Enjoy learning the techniques of hand reflexology and don't worry if your initial efforts seem slow or awkward for you will progress rapidly and develop your own unique style. Be prepared to be amazed at the results you achieve with this most intriguing of therapies. Whether you have a specific health problem you wish to treat, or you are just looking for a way to relieve the stresses and strains of everyday life and keep fit and healthy, reflexology is for you!

1 | AN EXPLANATION OF HAND REFLEXOLOGY

What is hand reflexology?

It is a simple, natural, non-invasive method of applying gentle pressure to the different surfaces of the hands using your fingers and thumbs. Our hands can be seen as a mirror image or a mini-map of the body. All the structures and organs – indeed even our life history – are reflected in miniature on the various parts of the hands. The health of the right side of the body is reflected in the right hand whereas the left side of the body in mirrored in the left hand. There is a reflex area for each individual part of the body. By stimulating these reflexes the natural healing forces are awakened, blockages are released and harmony and health are restored. Reflexology facilitates healing not only on a physical and emotional level but also on a spiritual level.

What are the benefits?

Hand reflexology offers a wide range of benefits, both physiological as well as psychological, for all the systems of the body. It:

■ Reduces stress and tension. Most of the illnesses that we suffer from are induced, or at least aggravated, by the stressful lives that we lead. As the stress is released symptoms such as headaches, irritable bowel syndrome and insomnia are relieved or may even disappear.

■ Induces a deep sense of relaxation. Once relaxed, body, mind and spirit are provided with optimum conditions for healing.

■ Revitalizes energy. The majority of people feel tired all the time or slightly under par. Very few of us jump out of bed in the morning raring to go! Hand reflexology can bring back that vitality and zest for life.

■ Stimulates mental function. Hand reflexology is excellent for improving concentration and stimulating creativity and new ideas. Try it when your brain feels sluggish or maybe if you are feeling indecisive!

■ Detoxifies the body. Impurities and toxins impair the functioning of our bodies. We clog ourselves up with junk food, too much tea and coffee, too little water and we forget to exercise properly. Why not combine a healthy lifestyle and a spring-clean of your body with the help of hand reflexology?

■ Balances the emotions. Hand reflexology can have a profound effect on the emotions. Fears and frustrations can be released, mood swings may be reduced, confidence is boosted, depression is lifted and generally individuals feel much more fulfilled and positive about life. You will feel much stronger emotionally (as well as physically) and will therefore be able to cope with the pressures of life much more readily, enabling you to take more control of your life. As you begin to think in a much more positive way you will find yourself attracting opportunities, thus creating room for personal development and transformation.

■ Helps to balance the systems of the body.

Circulatory system
Hand reflexology improves the blood flow to every part of the body bringing essential nutrients and oxygen to the cells. Blood pressure can be balanced and the strain on the heart may be reduced.

Digestive system
Indigestion, colic, constipation, irritable bowel syndrome, diverticulitis, colitis and many other

049219.

digestive disorders can improve as the absorption of nutrients becomes more efficient.

Genito–urinary system
Cystitis, bladder problems such as incontinence, kidney disorders and fluid retention can all be treated.

Lymphatic system
This system plays an important part in the body's defence against infection and disease. A sluggish lymphatic system can be activated.

Musculo-skeletal system
Aches and pains whether in the muscles or joints can be reduced. Sciatica, arthritis, rheumatism, gout and stiff joints will ease.

Nervous system
Anxiety, insomnia, headaches, migraine, neuralgia and stress-related disorders respond well to hand reflexology.

Reproductive system
Menstrual problems such as PMS, irregular, scanty, heavy menstruation, the menopause, infertility problems and lack of libido can be treated.

Respiratory system
Chest problems such as asthma, bronchitis, emphysema, excessive mucus and all ear, nose and throat problems may respond. Breathing deepens and mucus is eliminated with regular treatment.

Skin
Skin condition, texture and tone all improve greatly after hand reflexology. Problems such as acne, eczema, psoriasis and allergies can all be treated successfully.

■ Seeks out the cause of an illness. It is far better to seek the cause rather than simply palliating the systems. For instance, suppose that you are suffering from headaches. Hand reflexology would not just treat the reflex areas relating to the head – this would be a symptomatic treatment. The headaches could be due to sinus congestion, eyestrain, hormone problems, stress and anxiety, tension in the neck and shoulder area or could be digestive related. All these areas would be massaged to determine and treat the cause.

■ Does not have adverse reactions. Hand reflexology is a drug-free, non-invasive technique without side effects. A few minor reactions that are regarded as positive may occur either during or between treatments – these will be discussed later. It is a gentle, natural treatment unlike conventional drugs that can cause many side effects such as stomach problems, constipation and thrush. There are a few cases when extra care needs to be taken. Always refer to the contraindications on pages 28–9.

■ Prevents health problems from occurring. Regular reflexology treatment boosts immunity, raising levels of resistance to disease. By incorporating hand reflexology into your daily routine you will become far less susceptible to coughs and colds. When minor health problems do occur they can be nipped in the bud before they become serious.

■ Works well alongside orthodox medicine. More and more members of the medical profession are realizing the many benefits that reflexology can offer. It is used in many hospitals in all areas of care, including maternity, rheumatology, orthopaedics, the elderly, pain clinics, hospices, psychiatric care, paediatrics and intensive care. It can help reduce the number of medications needed considerably. However, drugs should *never* be withdrawn without the consent of the doctor.

> **CAUTION**
> Hand reflexology should never be used *instead* of orthodox medicine and the advice of a doctor should always be sought for persistent health problems. A reflexologist should *never* diagnose – this is the prerogative of a doctor. Reflexologists do not propose to cure, make no promises and do not give false hope.

Hand versus foot reflexology

Traditionally foot reflexology is used more frequently by reflexologists than hand reflexology, since some consider the feet to be more sensitive to treatment than the hands. However, it is becoming evident that, if used correctly, hand reflexology can achieve equal or even better results than foot reflexology.

Hand reflexology has many advantages:

- It can be carried out almost anywhere at any time. While travelling on a bus, train or plane; if you are queuing at the shops or waiting at the doctor, dentist or hairdresser; when you are relaxing in your lunch hour or tea break or watching television.
- It is easy to practise on yourself as well as on others. The hands are very accessible and can be treated as often as is necessary. It is an ideal form of self-treatment.
- It can reinforce the work carried out by a professional reflexologist, thus accelerating recovery time.
- If, for instance, a foot is sprained or fractured, then working the hand/hands becomes a necessity as foot reflexology is contraindicated.
- If the feet are infected or if parts of the feet are afflicted with, for example, a common fungal infection such as athlete's foot (tinea pedis) or a viral infection such as a verruca, it is advisable to treat the hands instead.
- When a foot or part of a foot is inflamed the hands should be treated. There may be gout in the big toe,

which can be excruciating, a painful bunion or severe rheumatoid arthritis.

- If a foot has been amputated then hand reflexology is the natural option.
- If a person is too shy or embarrassed to expose their feet or is fearful that the treatment will be too ticklish, then hand reflexology is advantageous.

How does it work?

It is not fully understood how and why reflexology works. However, the healing power of reflexology is proven every day. There are several theories, and it is my opinion that all of these contain an element of truth – no one single theory can totally satisfy my sceptical mind. There is a great deal in this world that cannot be entirely explained. The fact that reflexology does work is proof enough for me of its enormous worth! The three main theories are as follows:

1 **Theory of crystalline deposits**

 Many reflexologists believe that if the body's metabolism is not functioning properly then waste products, such as uric acid and excess calcium, are deposited in the hands and feet. These crystalline deposits may be dispersed by the application of reflexology and eliminated.

2 **Nerve ending theory**

 There are thousands of nerve endings in the hands and feet that have connections with many parts of the body. It is postulated that stimulation of these nerve endings results in responses elsewhere in the body.

3 **Theory of energy flow**

 If optimum health is to be maintained it is vital that the energy or *chi* flows freely. Any blockages in this flow will result in dis-ease and ill health. By massaging the reflex zones, blockages are released and the *chi* can flow freely enabling healing to take place. Reflexologists believe that there are ten energy zones, which will be discussed later.

Brief history of reflexology

Reflexology has been practised in various forms for thousands of years by many diverse cultures the world over. The techniques were passed down from generation to generation. The Egyptians, Chinese, Indians and Native Americans all realized the importance of hand and foot reflexology.

It is fascinating that in ancient Egypt during the mummification process the soles of the feet were removed in order to free the soul from the confines of the earth plane. In Saqqara, in the tomb of the Egyptian physician, Ankmahor, an illustration dating back to 2300 BC depicts treatment of the hands and feet actually being performed.

Dr William Fitzgerald (1872–1942), the American physician, is seen as the father of reflexology. He claimed that applying pressure to key points on the hands and feet could result in physiological changes in other parts of the body. He published a book in 1917 with his colleague, Dr Edwin Bowers, entitled *Zone Therapy. Relieving Pain at Home*.

Dr Joseph Shelby Riley took on board his theories. He is renowned for introducing Eunice Ingham, a physiotherapist, to the ideas of zone therapy. Eunice Ingham (1879–1974) is acknowledged as the 'mother' of reflexology. She dedicated her life to the practice and teaching of reflexology and mapped out the entire body on the hands and feet. She died in 1974 but reflexology has continued to flourish and develop, gaining worldwide recognition.

Principles of hand reflexology

The hand is divided into longitudinal (vertical) and transverse (horizontal) zones.

The longitudinal (vertical) zones

The body can be divided into ten longitudinal zones that run the entire length of the body from the tips of the toes to the head, out to the fingertips and visa versa. If an imaginary line is drawn through the centre of the body, there are five situated on the right side of this midline and five on the left.

- **Zone 1** runs from the big toe, up the leg and centre of the body to the head and down to the thumb.
- **Zone 2** extends from the second toe up to the head and down to the index finger.
- **Zone 3** goes from the third toe up to the head and then down to the third finger.
- **Zone 4** runs from the fourth toe up to the head and down to the fourth finger.
- **Zone 5** extends from the fifth toe up to the head and then down to the little finger.

Why not try tracing these zones on your own body?

Within these zones lie all the organs and structures of the body. All the points within one zone are related to each other. Therefore if a reflex point is stimulated in Zone 3 in the hand, all the structures in Zone 3 throughout the body will be affected.

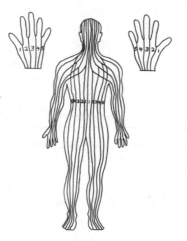

Figure 1.1   The ten longitudinal (vertical) zones

The transverse/horizontal zones

The three transverse or horizontal zones enable us to map the hands even more precisely.

The first transverse zone, otherwise known as the **diaphragm line** is located just below the padded area beneath the fingers. It is found about 2.5 cm (1″) down from the join of the index finger to the hand. All the structures above the diaphragm on the body are mirrored above this line. Therefore reflexes to areas such as the face, sinuses, ears, eyes, teeth, throat, head, brain, neck and shoulders would be found above the diaphragm line.

The second transverse zone is also known as the **waistline**. It runs from the base of the thumb (where the bottom of the thumb joins the hand) across to the other side of the hand.

The third transverse zone, known as the **pelvic line**, circles the wrist.

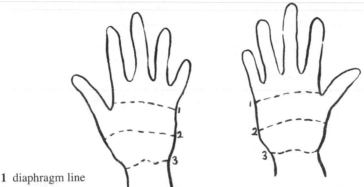

1 diaphragm line
2 waist line
3 pelvic line

Figure 1.2   The transverse horizontal zones

The hands are a mirror of the body. The right side of the body is represented in the right hand whereas the left side of the body is reflected in the left. Paired organs, such as the kidneys or lungs, will be located in both hands – the right kidney/lung in the right hand and the left kidney/lung in the left hand.

Both the transverse zones and the horizontal zones enable us to pinpoint accurately the reflexes on the hands.

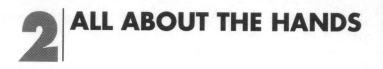

2 | ALL ABOUT THE HANDS

The structure of the hands

Each hand and wrist is made up of 27 bones. These bones comprise eight carpals, five metacarpals and 14 phalanges.

Carpals (these bones make up the wrist or carpus)

The carpals are arranged in two rows of four and are bound together closely and firmly by ligaments. They are named in Latin according to their shape. The first row nearest the metacarpals (known as the distal row) comprises:

- Trapezium
- Trapezoid
- Capitate
- Hamate.

The second row (known as the proximal row) nearest the bones of the forearm (i.e. the radius and ulna) comprises:

- Scaphoid
- Lunate
- Triquetral/Triquetrum
- Pisiform.

Metacarpals

These five bones form the skeleton of the palm of the hand. The heads of these bones make up the knuckles.

Phalanges

These are the finger and thumb bones. The thumb has only two phalanges, whereas the fingers each have three phalanges.

The bones of the hand and wrist are held in place by numerous muscles, tendons and ligaments.

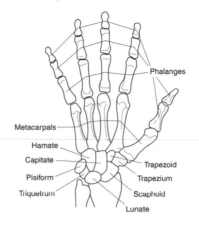

Figure 2.1   The bony structure of the hands

The human hand is quite remarkable. Its delicate movements allow grasping and fine movements. Only in humans can the thumb be brought into opposition with each of the other fingers. The hands are very sensitive and are capable of perceiving the lightest of touch, changes in temperature and of measuring thickness.

Aspects of the hands

It is important to familiarize yourself with the different surfaces of the hands. This will enable you to carry out a hand reflexology treatment easily and without confusion. The areas you need to be clear about are:

- ■ the tips of the fingers
- ■ the back of the hand (dorsal aspect)
- ■ the palm of the hand (palmar side)
- ■ the outside of the hand (lateral aspect/little finger side)
- ■ the inside of the hand (medial aspect/thumb side).

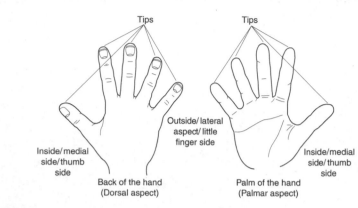

Figure 2.2   Aspects of the hand

Problems affecting the hands and wrists

Carpal Tunnel Syndrome

Symptoms

Pain, tingling, numbness and even weakness in the hand, especially in the thumb, index and middle fingers. Pain may also radiate to the elbow. It is usually worse at night and can be relieved by raising the arm or placing the hand in cold water.

Causes

This condition arises from compression on the median nerve as it passes into the hand through a narrow channel (the carpal tunnel) at the base of the palm of the hand. It is frequent among workers using computer keyboards, people who use their hands a lot and in women aged 30–60. It also occurs fairly frequently in pregnancy; while taking oral contraceptives; during the menopause; and in men and women who suffer from rheumatoid arthritis, gout or thyroid problems.

Treatment

Various treatments such as rest, splints, diuretics and local steroid injections are administered. As a very last resort the ligament is surgically cut to relieve pressure on the nerve. Hand reflexology can help this condition considerably by easing pressure on the nerve and providing pain relief.

Raynaud's disease

Symptoms

Tingling, numbness and burning is experienced in the fingers (and toes sometimes). When exposed to the cold, the fingers turn white due to lack of blood caused by spasm in the small arteries; the digits then become blue due to lack of oxygen; finally they turn red, as the blood flow is re-established.

Causes

There is no known cause but the condition is sometimes familial. For reasons unknown the small arteries which supply blood to the fingers contract suddenly when exposed to the cold, resulting in restricted blood flow to the area.

Treatment

A sufferer of Raynaud's disease is advised to keep the hands as warm as possible and to stop smoking. Vasodilator drugs are sometimes prescribed. Regular hand reflexology treatment is excellent for this condition. Sufferers can treat themselves daily for best results.

Dupuytren's contracture

Symptoms

A small, hard tender nodule on the palm of the hand is often the first sign. This gradually becomes a band of thickened tissue and leads to contraction of the palmar fascia and puckering of the skin. The fingers start to contract and may become fixed in a bent position. The ring finger is the most frequently affected, followed by the little and middle fingers. The flexion can become so severe that the fingernails dig into the palm.

Causes

This condition primarily affects men over the age of 40. In some cases there may be a hereditary tendency. Sometimes it is found in alcoholics and it can be triggered or aggravated by trauma.

Treatment

Surgical treatment is usually advised but may not be successful. Hand reflexology can alleviate this condition. Self-treatment over the thickened band of tissue several times a day and mobilizing the finger joints produces excellent results.

Tenosynovitis

Symptoms

Tendons in the hand and wrist are most commonly affected. Due to inflammation of the synovial sheaths that protect the tendon, the area over the affected tendon becomes painful, tender and swollen. It will be painful to move the affected wrist. When you move the wrist there is usually a grating sensation called crepitus.

Causes

It can be caused by a job that involves repetitive movements.

Treatment

The hand and wrist may be immobilized in a splint for a few weeks. Anti-inflammatory drugs may be prescribed. Do not practise reflexology over the affected area while it is inflamed. After the swelling has subsided and the tenosynovitis has settled down, gentle hand reflexology can help to mobilize the wrist.

Trigger finger/thumb

Symptoms

The ring or the middle finger is the most frequently affected. The finger involved is locked in a bent position. When the finger does straighten, an audible snap is heard.

Causes

It is caused by a nodule in a tendon in the palm near the head of the metacarpal. The nodule is too big to enter the tendon sheath easily when the person tries to straighten the finger from a bent position.

Treatment

Cortisone injection or surgery to widen the opening of the sheath. Gentle hand reflexology can help to alleviate this condition, provided it is started early on and administered regularly.

Ganglion

Symptoms

Ganglions are extremely common in the hand and wrist, particularly on the dorsum. A lump varying in size from the size of a small pea to a golf ball is visible. Although unsightly, ganglions are usually painless. Sometimes full movement may be impaired and occasionally they may become painful.

Causes

A ganglion is a well-defined fluid-filled swelling associated with the synovial sheath of a tendon. It may appear for no apparent reason. It can be associated with overuse, or may be caused by an injury to the tendons on the back of the joint.

Treatment

Usually no treatment is prescribed as they may disappear spontaneously. However, there are some instances when they need to be excised. Regular hand reflexology over the site can be used to speed up the disappearance of the ganglion.

Osteoarthritis

Symptoms

A very common joint disease occurring after middle age, especially in weight-bearing joints such as hips and knees, causing pain, stiffness and loss of mobility. Hard nodules, known as Heberden's nodes, may be visible on the finger joints.

Causes

A degenerative disorder associated with wear and tear. Injuries earlier on in life may increase the chances of developing arthritis in that particular joint.

Treatment

Analgesics (and corticosteroid injections) are administered to control the pain. Hand reflexology is invaluable in cases of arthritis as it can help to lessen the stiffness in the joints, thereby improving and maintaining mobility.

Rheumatoid arthritis

Symptoms

Rheumatoid arthritis very frequently affects the hands and wrists. The joints become very swollen, tender, red, warm, painful and stiff. It can become difficult to grip objects and the hands may become very deformed with deviation of the fingers. Joint thickening and muscle wasting are further symptoms of this condition.

Causes

Rheumatoid arthritis is an autoimmune disorder whereby the immune system attacks its own tissue. It usually starts in middle age but can affect children and is more common in women. There is no known cause although there may be an inherited tendency.

Treatment

Painkillers and anti-inflammatory drugs are prescribed. In severe cases surgery may be performed to replace destroyed joints. Hand reflexology is excellent here. It can help to mobilize the joints and provide much needed pain relief.

Warts

Symptoms

A very common, contagious, harmless skin growth affecting only the top layer of skin. They are firm, round or irregular, flesh-coloured or brown often with a rough surface. Sometimes black dots can be seen, which are capillaries that have become clotted as a result of the rapid skin growth of the wart.

Causes

Warts are caused by the humanpapilomavirus (HPV). They are contagious.

Treatment

They usually disappear naturally. They can be treated by applying a wart-removing liquid, liquid nitrogen which freezes the wart or by laser treatment. Cover up a wart with a plaster before commencing a hand reflexology treatment. Apply neat essential oil of tea tree to the wart several times a day on a cotton bud for a couple of weeks to destroy it.

Fingernail problems

Paronychia

This is a common skin infection occurring between the base of the nail and the cuticle. It is characterized by inflammation, swelling and sometimes tenderness. Paronychia is most prevalent among women, especially those who have poor circulation and spend a lot of time with their hands in the water.

Spoon-shaped nails (koilonychias)

The nails are dry, brittle and thin and eventually become spoon-shaped. It may be caused by injury to the nail and is sometimes seen in iron-deficiency anaemia.

Clubbing of the nails

In early clubbing the angle between nail and nail base straightens out. The nail base feels springy. In late clubbing the base of the nail becomes visibly swollen and the fingernails curve. Clubbing is associated with some chronic lung diseases such as lung cancer, bronchiectasis and lung abscess.

Oriental diagnosis

Oriental diagnosis can be used to detect many disorders and can even pinpoint potential problems before they arise. The principles behind oriental diagnosis were developed and preserved in Japan, China, Korea and India for many centuries among religious, cultural and philosophical traditions.

The hands can reveal both recent and present physical and mental conditions. The *palm* of the hand reflects the physical condition whereas the *fingers* reveal the mental tendencies.

The finger

Each finger is said to correspond to a part of the body:

Thumb – corresponds to the lungs and their functions
Index finger – represents the large intestines and their functions
Middle finger – represents the heart and circulatory functions and reproductive functions
Ring finger – controls vitality, temperature and energy
Little finger – corresponds to the function of the heart (palm side) and the small intestine (back of the hand).

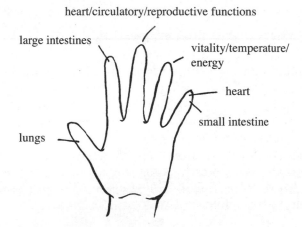

Figure 2.3   Correlation between the fingers and organs and the systems of the body

Thick, strong fingers with a well-developed bone structure indicate a strong physical constitution. Thin, long fingers show a more mental and spiritual nature with an orientation towards the arts. Musicians and other creative people often have these types of fingers. When the hand is fully stretched if the fingers can curve backwards this shows a greater mental and spiritual capacity. If the fingers tend to curve forwards this indicates physical strength and mental rigidity.

The fingertips

Shape

The tips of the fingers can reveal constitution and character:

Square fingertips show a character that is physically active, determined and possibly aggressive.

Round fingertips show a happy, active, energetic and positive character who is understanding and sympathetic.

Pointed, narrow fingertips show a tendency to be physically weaker with a sensitive and artistic nature.

Expanded, swollen fingertips reveals a more self-centred, aggressive and argumentative personality.

Condition

Hard, flaky skin on the fingertips indicates physical and mental rigidity.

Soft peeling skin on the fingertips shows emotional irritability and mental sensitivity.

Cracked, split fingertips show that the circulatory, excretory and reproductive systems are not functioning harmoniously. There may be impotence or frigidity.

White fatty skin may indicate mucus accumulating in the lungs and disorders in the digestive system.

Red or purple fingertips can reveal nervousness, irritability, over-sensitivity or depression.

The nails

Colour

Pinkish, red nails reveal general good health, both physically and mentally.

Whitish nails show under-active blood circulation and may be indicative of anaemia. People in good health do not usually have this whitish colour in the nails.

Shape

Square stocky nails show a tendency towards physical activity but mental inflexibility.

Oblong nails reveal a more physically and mentally balanced constitution. There may be a slight rigidity.

Oval nails may show a weaker physical constitution but an active mind and emotional sensitivity.

Texture

Thick/hard nails show vitality and physical and mental strength.

Soft/thin nails reveal a weaker physical constitution but someone who is mentally active and sensitive.

Nail Variations

Vertical ridges show imbalanced nutrition. There will often be fatigue.

Horizontal indentations reveal changes in diet. If there are several indentations this shows that more than one dietary change has taken place. It takes about 6–9 months for adult nails to grow, so it is possible to work out exactly when the change occurred.

Split/uneven nails shows a nutritional imbalance. The nervous system is under pressure and the reproductive system may be functioning abnormally.

Larger white moons at the base of the nails tend to reveal a physically active person.

Small moons reveal a mentally active person with a slow metabolism.

During childhood and adolescence everyone has moons, but these tend to disappear during old age.

3 | **PREPARATION FOR HAND REFLEXOLOGY**

It is not necessary to have any expensive or complicated equipment to carry out hand reflexology. All that is needed is a willing pair of hands, your intuition and the desire to help others. Although hand reflexology can be carried out successfully anywhere, the ideal environment is one that promotes peace and relaxation. A few simple steps to create the right ambience will ensure that the recipient receives maximum benefit from the treatment.

General preparation

Disconnect the telephone or take it off the hook and tell your family, if necessary, that you are carrying out a treatment and do not want to be disturbed. Warm the room prior to the treatment to encourage feelings of deep relaxation and security. Lighting should be soft and subdued. Bright lights are not conducive to relaxation. Use a dimmer switch if you have one, or even better, light some candles. Particularly soothing colours are pastel shades such as lavender, pale pink, blue or green. Burn some essential oils. Aromatherapy oils are highly therapeutic for body, mind and spirit and are an excellent way to enhance your treatment (for more information on the healing art of aromatherapy see *Teach Yourself Aromatherapy* by the same author).

Some suggested oils are:

Sedative oils to calm the mind and encourage sleep:

- Chamomile
- Clary sage
- Geranium
- Jasmine

- Lavender
- Marjoram
- Neroli
- Rose
- Sandalwood
- Ylang Ylang.

Uplifting oils to ease depression and encourage positivity:

- Bergamot
- Grapefruit
- Jasmine
- Lime
- Mandarin
- Palmarosa.

Life-changing oils to enable you to move on and let go of the past:

- Cedarwood
- Cypress
- Frankincense
- Linden blossom
- Rosewood.

Stimulating oils to invigorate body and mind, improve concentration and memory and strengthen the immune system:

- Basil
- Black pepper
- Ginger
- Lemon
- Lemongrass
- Orange
- Peppermint
- Rosemary.

Detoxifying oils to assist elimination of waste products (mind, body and spirit):

- Cypress
- Fennel

- Grapefruit
- Juniper
- Lemon
- Rosemary.

Aphrodisiac oils to heal relationships and develop sensuality:

- Jasmine
- Neroli
- Rose
- Sandalwood
- Ylang Ylang.

A small inexpensive clay burner is ideal for diffusing your essential oils. Simply put a few teaspoons of water into the bowl on the top of your oil burner and sprinkle a few drops of your favourite essential oils into it.

Put some fresh flowers in the room to enhance the ambience and place a few crystals around the room. A piece of pink rose quartz encourages love and peace and purple amethyst absorbs any negativity. Blue stones such as blue lace agate and blue calcite are also very relaxing.

Play some music to relax body, mind and spirit and to keep conversation to a minimum. New Age music is particularly therapeutic. Some enjoy Gregorian chants, dolphin or whale music, Buddhist chants or sounds such as the wind and the sea. It is entirely up to the individual, as some people will enjoy silence during their treatment.

Have several pillows ready to ensure the comfort of both you and the recipient and towels or a blanket may be needed to make the recipient feel secure, warm and relaxed. Place some purified water in the room for use at the end of the reflexology session to flush away the toxins and if you intend to massage the hands with an aromatherapy blend at the end of the treatment to enhance the effect of reflexology, have your oils ready (see Chapter 8 for suggestions).

Personal preparation

Remove all jewellery from your hands since rings, bracelets and watches can all scratch the receiver and wear comfortable, loose-fitting clothes so that you can relax and move around easily. Clip your nails closely to avoid digging them into the recipient and do not wear strong perfumes or eat highly spiced foods (unless they have!), as this can be off-putting if the smell is unpleasant to the receiver. Wash your hands and check that your nails are scrupulously clean.

Finally, spend time relaxing yourself prior to the session. Close your eyes, take a few deep breaths and as you breathe out feel the tension floating out of your body. If you have any tightness in the neck and shoulders, gently breathe into these areas allowing the tension to dissolve away. If you have any negative thoughts, allow them to melt away. This will enable the healing energies to flow through you and allow you to be guided by your intuition during the treatment.

Preparation of the receiver

Explain briefly to the receiver what reflexology is (see page 1). If he/she knows what to expect then there will be no need for any apprehension. Position the receiver in one of the following ways ready for the treatment:

Laying down

A professional reflexologist will have a massage couch but this is not essential if you are working on your family, friends or yourself. A bed, reclining chair or a sun-lounger is quite acceptable if the recipient wishes to lie down. You can also create a firm, well-padded working surface on the floor by placing a thick duvet, several blankets or a sleeping bag on the floor. Place pillows/cushions under the receiver's head for comfort and to enable you to observe any facial expressions. Also place one under the knees to take the pressure off the lower back and one under the hand that you have decided to treat first. Cover the recipient with a sheet, blanket or towel depending upon the temperature and make sure that they are comfortable and relaxed. If they are wearing any tight, restrictive clothing, such as ties or belts, then these may be loosened.

Sitting down

The receiver may also sit facing you with his/her hand resting on a small table or stool. This should be covered with a pillow/cushion with a small towel placed on top. You can also place one or two pillows on your knees covered with a towel and rest the receiver's hand on your lap. Personally, I find it most beneficial for the receiver to lie down. This seems to be most conducive for healing and relaxation. Whichever position you choose make sure that you are comfortable too! Place a swivel chair or stool so that the receiver's hand is readily accessible. It is vital that you feel relaxed so that the energy flows freely and you are able to detect any hand reflexes that need to be balanced.

Examining the hands

Healthy hands that are a good colour with unblemished skin and good muscle tone indicate a healthy person! The hands should be pleasantly warm, but not moist and clammy and fingernails should be strong. They should also be supple, relaxed and mobile. It never ceases to amaze me what a physical examination can reveal about a person's health and personality. Look for the following:

Skin condition

Are there any areas of hard or thin flaccid skin? Is the skin dry, cracked, flaking or peeling?

Areas of hard skin on the hands are sometimes a protective mechanism to stop one from getting hurt or may hide one's true feelings. They can also be indicative of resistance and lack of flexibility.

Dry, flaking skin can appear during periods of change. The body is letting go of the past and preparing for the new. It can also suggest emotional vulnerability.

Are there any blisters due to constant friction? Perhaps an aspect of their life is causing this friction.

Is there any infection on the hands?

Are there any warts?

Can you see any cuts, scars, spots or rashes?

Is there a ganglion?

Are the hands firm or flabby?

Is there any puffiness in the fingers or swelling around the wrists?

Skin temperature

Are the hands overly warm, clammy and moist?

Are they very cold?

Clammy hands may be an indication of nervousness or may be due to excessive toxicity. Cold hands show that the circulation is poor and sometimes reveals that the recipient finds it difficult to let go and express him/herself.

Skin colour

The hands may be all sorts of colours – pale, white, red, yellow, purple or mottled. White hands may indicate tiredness and exhaustion; red hands anger and frustration; yellow, purple or mottled hands reveal toxins in the body and emotional hurts.

Nails

Are the nails a healthy pink or white, or are they tinged with blue reflecting an under active circulation? Are they split, flaked, broken, hardened, ridged or a strange shape? (Refer to oriental diagnosis on page 20 for explanations.)

Bony structure

Is there any arthritis in the hands distorting the shape and decreasing mobility in the fingers? Are any fingers gnarled or locked in a bent position? Sometimes this may reveal inflexibility and a dislike for change.

As you can see the hands reveal all sorts of past experiences and emotions as well as physical problems.

The *site* of the abnormality, whatever it may be, is very important from a reflexology point of view. For instance, hard skin or a wart down the outer aspect of the thumb will reflect a neck problem, since this is where the reflex area for the neck is located. Deviation or abnormalities of the fingers can indicate problems with the sinuses or teeth. Puffiness around the wrist reveals a clogged up lymphatic system, since this is where the reflexes to the pelvic lymphatics are located.

Contraindications to hand reflexology

Hand reflexology is a very safe and natural therapy. It should always be performed gently and should *never* be painful. It should be an extremely relaxing and blissful experience. However, there are a limited number of cases when advice should be sought prior to the treatment, or extra care needs to be taken. If you are at all unsure then please seek the advice of a medically qualified doctor or a professional reflexologist.

When not to perform hand reflexology

Never treat patients:

- If the receiver is suffering from deep vein thrombosis or phlebitis, as the clot could dislodge.
- Immediately after surgery due to the risk of thrombosis, until the doctor has pronounced complete recovery. Research shows that reflexology accelerates recovery time but only a very light treatment is given during the initial stages.
- If the receiver has a contagious skin disease such as scabies, ringworm or chickenpox. You do not want to aggravate the condition or spread it to yourself or others.
- If the receiver has a fever – wait until it has subsided. A hand reflexology treatment releases toxins into the system and as the body is already fighting off toxins it has enough to contend with.

Exercise caution

You should be aware of the following:

- Do not use hand reflexology over the reproductive areas during pregnancy. Take particular care during the first three months. If there is a history of miscarriage then consult a fully qualified reflexologist.
- Take care when treating a diabetic. Use less pressure as the skin may be thinner, more fragile, bruise more easily and is slower to heal. Do not press on the pancreas area if you are not a qualified reflexologist.
- When treating people with heart problems, avoid the heart reflex if a pacemaker has been fitted and take care if the recipient has cardiac problems.
- Calluses, nodules, areas of thickened skin – use gentle pressure if they are painful.
- Cuts and warts – cover them up during the treatment.
- Bruises and any other tender, painful areas – use very gentle pressure
- When treating the elderly, perform a light treatment as the skin may be thinner and conditions such as arthritis and osteoporosis (fragile bones) may be present. If a joint is very inflamed or painful then take extra
  special care.
- When treating children, a light pressure is required, and the younger they are the shorter the treatment. Usually 10–15 minutes will suffice.
- Take care when working on the terminally ill. Gentle pressure can be extremely beneficial, helping to relieve pain, relax, uplift and improving elimination.
- Epilepsy – use gentle presuure over the head and brain areas.

REMEMBER!

■ *Never* diagnose, as reflexology is not a diagnostic tool.
■ Do not promise to cure or give false hope.

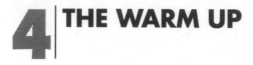

4 | THE WARM UP

Relaxation techniques are always used at the beginning of a reflexology session to:

- help put both of you at ease
- establish a sense of trust
- dispel any worries that the recipient might have
- enable you to gauge how much pressure the recipient will need in the treatment
- increase flexibility in the hands.

These relaxation techniques will also be used during the reflexology routine to disperse any toxins that have been released from the reflex areas, to soothe and relax, and to loosen and mobilize the hands further. At the end of the session they can be used as a 'dessert' to bring your treatment to a close.

You may use as many of my suggested movements as you wish. It is not essential to perform them in any particular order and they can be adapted to suit the recipient's needs. Be creative and intuitive – if it feels good it must be having a beneficial effect.

Technique 1

Greeting the hand

Take hold of the recipient's hand and clasp it gently between both your hands. Hold it for about a minute or two and notice how relaxed you both become. This initial contact will enable you to tune in to the receiver and notice any sensations that you may feel or heat or tingling as the healing forces are mobilized.

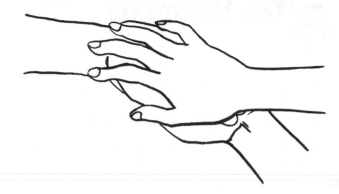

Figure 4.1   Greeting the hand

Technique 2

Stroking the hand

Supporting the receiver's wrist with the palm downwards with one hand, gently stroke up to the top of the hand. Glide lightly back using no pressure. Repeat this movement several times and then turn his/her hand over and repeat on the palm of the hand. If you wish to make your stroking firmer then you may use the heel of your hand. Notice how warm the hand becomes as the blood flow increases and the recipient relaxes.

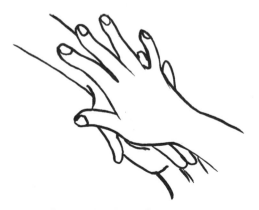

Figure 4.2   Stroking the hand

Technique 3

Opening the hand

Take the palm uppermost in both of yours. With your thumbs parallel and touching in the centre of the recipient's palm, slide your thumbs gently out to the sides. Repeat this movement several times in rows to gradually open up the palm. You may turn the hand over and repeat these movements on the dorsum (top) of the hand.

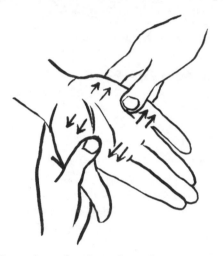

Figure 4.3   Opening the hand

Technique 4

Knuckling the palm/metacarpal kneading

Make a gentle fist with one hand while supporting the receiver's hand, palm uppermost, with your other hand. Place your fist on to the palm and make gentle circular movements to loosen up the numerous muscles, joints and tendons.

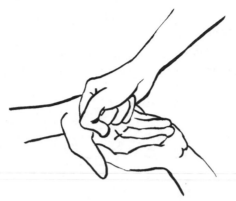

Figure 4.4   Knuckling the palm/metacarpal kneading

Technique 5

Circling the palm

With the palm uppermost interlock both your little fingers with the receiver's hand. Place both your thumbs on the palm and using small, outward circular movements work the whole of the palm of the hand. This technique helps to soften and relax the tissues.

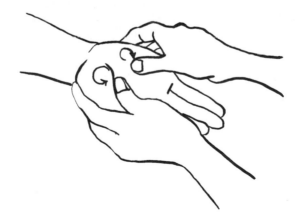

Figure 4.5   Circling the palm

Technique 6

Loosening the wrist

Gently holding the receiver's hand between your fingers, use your thumbs to work in small circles gently all around the wrist.

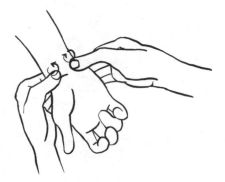

Figure 4.6   Loosening the wrist

Technique 7

Moving the wrist

Interlock your fingers with the receiver's fingers. Gently and slowly move the wrist backwards and forwards, side-to-side, clockwise and anti-clockwise. This movement is marvellous for keeping the wrists supple and mobile. Wonderful for arthritis!

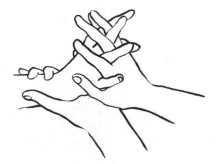

Figure 4.7   Moving the wrist

Technique 8

Loosening and moving the fingers and thumbs

Gently grasp the receiver's wrist to provide support. Using your thumb and index finger gently stretch and circle each finger individually. You may also flex and extend each of the finger joints for extra flexibility.

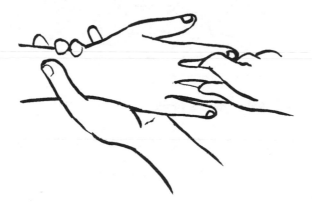

Figure 4.8   Loosening and moving the fingers and thumbs

Technique 9

Solar plexus release

Place your thumb onto the solar plexus reflex, which is located almost in the centre of the palm. Press gently and slowly into the area. As you do this you may notice the receiver's breathing begin to deepen as they completely let go of any residual tension.

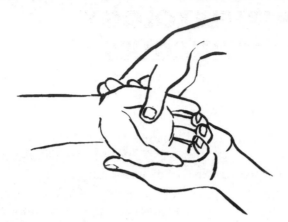

Figure 4.9   Solar plexus release

To complete your relaxation, gently stroke the receiver's hand as in Technique 1 but using a feather light touch. Now practise these techniques on the receiver's other hand until you feel confident that you have mastered them.

5 | REFLEXOLOGY TECHNIQUES

In this chapter you are going to learn the main techniques that you will be using to work on the reflex areas of the hands.

As you practise these techniques it is important to be sensitive to the needs of the recipient. The amount of pressure required varies enormously from one individual to another and you need to be able to adjust your pressure accordingly. The pressure should not be so gentle that the receiver feels a slight tickling sensation; it should be fairly firm but not painful. If the receiver flinches or tries to pull his/her hand away then you know that you need to reduce the pressure. Always ask for feedback.

It is often the case that physical, down-to earth, no-nonsense individuals seem to prcfcr a fairly firm pressure, whereas the more sensitive, spiritual souls favour a much lighter treatment.

Holding technique

It is vital to support the hands throughout the reflexology session. You need to have full control of the hands as you carry out your treatment and you should be able to reach and pinpoint all the reflex zones easily and accurately. The receiver should be able to see clearly everything that you are doing and if you support the hands correctly this will give him/her confidence and trust in your treatment.

Always avoid gripping the hands too tightly as you work on them. Also ensure that you are not pulling the skin taut, as this will create discomfort. Be aware of any painful joints or tender areas of the hand that you have observed during your physical examination (see pages 26–7). A therapeutic and sensitive touch will ensure a successful hand reflexology treatment.

An ideal holding position is to rest the receiver's hand, palm uppermost, gently in the palm of your hand.

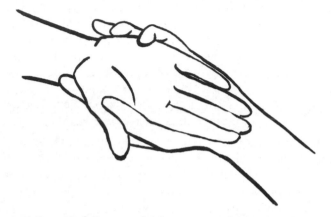

Figure 5.1   Holding technique (working on the palm)

When you need to work on the dorsal side (top), simply support the receiver's wrist from underneath as if you are shaking their hand.

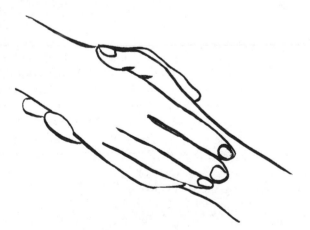

Figure 5.2   Holding technique (working on the top (dorsal) side)

Thumb walking/Caterpillar movements

This very important technique is used widely in reflexology and is particularly effective when working on large areas of the hand. As your thumb walks over the area being treated it should feel very relaxing to the receiver and as you perform this movement you will very quickly become aware of how much pressure the receiver is comfortable with. Try to exert a constant and steady pressure while contouring to the surfaces of the receiver's hands.

An excellent place to practise and master the caterpillar walking is on your forearm. At first your movements may feel clumsy or even jerky. But do not worry! Persevere and your thumb walking will soon feel smooth and even.

The outer edge of the thumb is used for this technique. If you are unsure about which is the inner and which is the outer edge of your thumb then place your hand palm downwards onto a flat surface such as a table. The tip of your thumb that is touching the surface is the *outer* edge and this will be the working area of your thumb.

To caterpillar walk bend the first joint of your thumb just *slightly* and then unbend the joint slightly. Notice that you have moved forward a little. Repeat this movement to walk right the way up your forearm. As you reach your elbow turn your hand round and walk from your elbow to your wrist. Practise on your other forearm so that you can caterpillar walk with both thumbs. Ensure that you are always moving *forwards*, as the thumb-walking technique is never performed backwards or sideways. Check that your thumb is only slightly bent it – should be neither too bent nor too straight. If your thumb is too bent you will dig your nail into the receiver's hand. It is *only* the first joint of the thumb that moves – the second joint of the thumb does not move but helps to create leverage. Although the entire hand participates in this movement the first joint of the thumb is the *only* moving part.

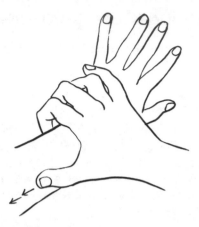

Figure 5.3   Thumbwalking technique on the forearm

After performing caterpillar walking on your forearm, practise it on the palm of you hand.

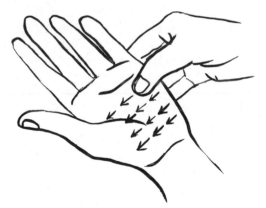

Figure 5.4   Caterpillar walking on the palm of the hand

You will soon feel confident to try thumb walking on a partner's hand. Do not worry if your thumbs feel slightly achy at first. This is unaccustomed exercise for your thumbs and they will quickly build up strength. Try thumb walking across the palm of the receiver's hand as well as from the base of the fingers to the wrist and from wrist to fingers. Now turn the hand over to walk across the hand and also down the hand in the troughs between the metacarpal bones.

Finger walking

If you have mastered thumb walking you will find finger walking easy! It is basically the same as thumb walking, except the first joint of the *index* finger (or fingers) is used. This technique is used in preference to thumb walking when working on bony or sensitive areas. An ideal place to practise is the dorsum (back) of your hand.

Finger walking may be practised with one finger or two or even more fingers. Practise *single finger walking* first. Place the tip of your index finger on the back of your hand and creep forwards across your hand taking the smallest possible steps.

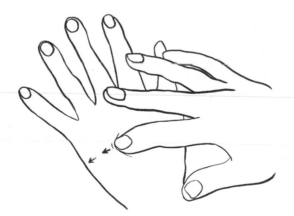

Figure 5.5   Single finger walking (own hand)

You may also try single finger walking working from the knuckles, down towards your wrist. Remember to use gentle pressure, as this technique is designed specifically for sensitive or bony areas where not much pressure is required.

Now try finger walking on a partner. Gently rest the receiver's hand, palm downwards, on the palm of your hand. Place the tip of your index finger just below one of their knuckles, bend the first joint of your index finger and off you go down towards the wrist!

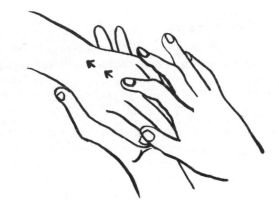

Figure 5.6   Single finger walking (on a partner)

Once you feel confident with single finger walking try *multiple finger walking*. Use your index finger to walk down the back of the receiver's hand. Now try using two, three, or even four fingers together. Much easier than you think, isn't it?

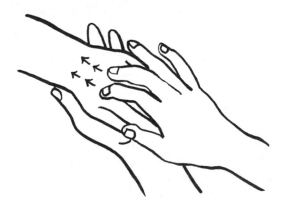

Figure 5.7   Multiple finger walking

You may rest the receiver's hand, palm downwards, and on the palm of your hand or as a variation place a fist under the palm of the receiver's hand to support it.

Pressure circles

This technique is usually performed using the pad of the thumb although occasionally the pad of a finger may be used. It is particularly indicated when sensitive areas are discovered on the hands. Gentle pressure circles allow any tenderness in an unbalanced reflex area to subside. This technique is very soothing and comforting.

Cup the receiver's hand, palm uppermost in your palm, gently press your thumb into an area and circle your thumb over it several times. After a few pressure circles any sensitivity should have diminished.

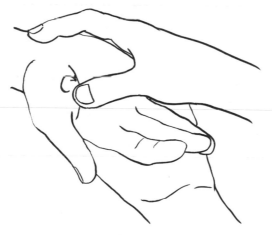

Figure 5.8 Pressure circles

Press and release

This technique is excellent for providing pain relief, for instance in cases of toothache or earache. It enables you to pinpoint specific areas and decrease sensitivity.

The tip of the thumb, finger or thumb and fingers(s) combined may be used. Do make sure that you do not dig your fingernails into the receiver's hand.

An excellent place to practise is in the webbing of the hand. Place the tip of the thumb in the webbing on top of the hand and the tip of the index finger on the webbing of the palm of the hand. Gently squeeze your finger and thumb towards each other – make sure that you do not pinch too hard! Hold your pressure for about 10–20 seconds and notice how any tenderness subsides.

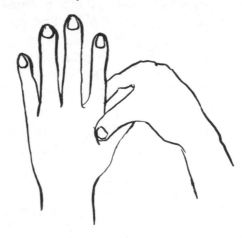

Figure 5.9   Press and release

Rotation on a point

Use this reflexology technique to pinpoint an area to be treated and rotate the hand around it. The pad of your thumb, index or other finger pinpoints the relevant reflex and remains stationary as the wrist is gently circled in both directions.

To practise this technique gently grasp the receiver's fingers, palm downward, with one hand. Use your chosen finger of your other hand to locate a relevant reflex point. Press into this point and keep your finger stationary as you circle the wrist with your supporting hand several times clockwise and anti-clockwise around the point.

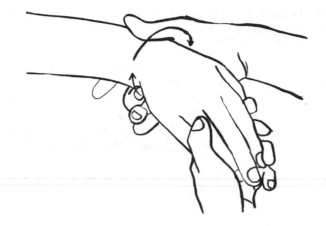

Figure 5.10   Rotation on a point

Hook in and back-up/pinpointing technique

Some reflexologists do not favour this technique but it is a classic technique and is marvellous for applying pressure to small reflex points that require great accuracy and which lie deep within the hand. The hook in and back-up technique is highly effective for balancing the pituitary gland in the thumb, which is of utmost importance when correcting hormonal imbalances.

Place the tip of your thumb onto a chosen point (try the centre of the first joint of the thumb as illustrated) and press into it (hook in) and then pull back across the point (back-up). Make sure that your thumbnail is not digging in. Some authorities liken this movement to a bee inserting its sting. A bee lands on a soft spot and backs its sting into your flesh. But do not worry, this technique will not be painful!

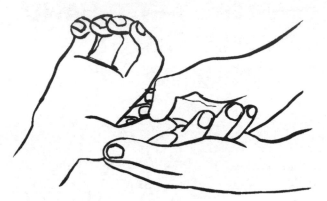

Figure 5.11   Hook in and back-up

Well done! You have now mastered the relaxation movements and all the reflexology techniques. You are now ready to carry out a complete hand reflexology treatment as outlined in the next chapter.

6 STEP-BY-STEP HAND REFLEXOLOGY SEQUENCE

This section will enable you to carry out a *complete* hand reflexology treatment. Detailed instructions and illustrations will guide you through each step of the treatment.

How long should a treatment take?

With practice, a treatment should take you about 30 minutes or maybe even less the more hands you work on. When working on frail or elderly individuals 15–20 minutes will suffice. A baby will require just a five-minute treatment consisting mostly of stroking movements and extremely gentle pressure on the reflex areas requiring attention. Longer is *not* more effective! If you work for too long you can over stimulate the reflexes and cause excessive elimination such as diarrhoea.

How many sessions will they need?

About four to six sessions performed on a weekly basis should be enough to keep the systems of the body in tip-top condition. This weekly interval between treatments allows time for self-healing to take place and enables any minor reactions to pass. Following the initial sessions, try to give a treatment about once a month. Of course if the receiver wants to be pampered you can safely treat every week!

If an acute problem such as a toothache, earache or sore throat arises, then the area(s) causing the problem may be treated several times a day to accelerate recovery. However, a *full* hand reflexology treatment should *not* be performed several times a day.

You may achieve amazing results after just one session – some individuals respond remarkably rapidly. Or you may need to wait several sessions for a response to your treatment. Always resist the temptation to give up – you will succeed with perseverance.

How much pressure should I use?

This depends entirely upon the individual, but generally your pressure should be firm but *not* painful. Ask the receiver for feedback so that you can adjust your pressure accordingly. A more physical, earthy person will usually favour a firm pressure whereas more sensitive individuals prefer a very light and gentle treatment. Always use gentle pressure on the elderly, diabetics, children and the terminally ill. Press lightly on tender, sensitive areas and use plenty of common sense.

What reactions can I expect?

All sorts of reactions may occur both during and in-between a reflexology treatment although it is impossible to predict which ones. However, rest assured that any change, whether physiological or psychological, should be seen as a positive sign and shows that your treatment is really working.

As you read through my list of reactions do not panic – it is impossible for the receiver to experience them all! Usually just one or two reactions occur and are short-lived, passing within 24 hours.

Possible reactions during hand reflexology

- A feeling of deep relaxation and tranquillity as the stress and tension subsides.
- Tingling sensations or warmth as blockages are released.
- Twitching or jerking as energy returns to previously deprived reflex areas.
- Deeper breathing and the desire to sleep.
- Changes in expression, such as frowning, when a sensitive area is palpated. A sharp pain is usually indicative of an acute problem whereas a dull pain is

often present when a chronic problem has existed for some time. The receiver will often smile as he/she slips into a state of bliss.

■ Noises such as sighing, laughing or crying.

■ Contraction of the muscles. For example, you may notice the shoulders or the neck move as you press the relevant reflex areas.

■ Runny nose, if the head zones are being worked on and are blocked.

■ Coughing as the chest reflexes are treated where there is congestion.

■ Gurgling noises as the colon is worked on.

■ The receiver may see beautiful colours such as blues, mauves and pink as the healing forces are mobilized.

■ A remembrance of past experiences.

Beware of a strong reaction!

It is highly unlikely that the following reaction will occur but I always think it is best to be prepared for everything. This will ensure that you stay calm and do not panic.

If the receiver starts to sweat excessively and begins to feel uneasy and possibly has palpitations, this is a sign that he/she has become over-stimulated. This is not necessarily your fault – the receiver may be overly sensitive or going through a particularly difficult, stressful period of his/her life. If you do not press too hard for long periods of time over sensitive reflex areas this should *never* occur.

However, if such a reaction should occur do *not* break off your treatment. Effleurage the hand gently and clasp it lightly between both your hands. Ask them to take a few deep breaths until the reaction subsides. If they wish to talk or cry then this should be encouraged as a release is taking place. Listen to them sympathetically without interrupting. If they do not wish to verbalize their feelings then respect their wishes. Offer them tissues if necessary, and a glass of water. Reassure them that this sort of reaction can occasionally happen but it is highly unlikely it will happen during their next treatment. Put your arm around them and give them a hug to offer comfort and reassurance. Encourage them to drink lots of water over the next few days to flush out the toxins.

Possible reactions between treatments

The receiver will find that he/she:

- Feels much more relaxed and able to cope with the pressures of everyday life.
- Thinks more clearly.
- Concentrates and focuses more easily.
- Feels more confident.
- Sleeps much better and awakens refreshed.
- Lives life to the full.
- Looks for the positive in everything.
- Feels revitalized and energized.
- Becomes much more patient and accommodating.
- Shows more compassion towards others.
- Needs to drink more water to flush away the toxins.

The following reactions between treatments shows that the body's self-healing mechanism has been awakened and that a process of purification has begun:

- Frequent dreaming as emotional baggage is cast aside.
- Increased skin activity leading to temporary rashes and pimples as irritations come to the surface.
- Increase in urination, which may be cloudy or unpleasant smelling as fears are released.
- Fever as the body raises its temperature to rid itself of physical and emotional toxins.
- Increase in bulk and volume of the stools and possibly even diarrhoea as unwanted pressures are let go of.
- Vaginal discharges as female issues are sorted out.
- Increase in perspiration as fear is washed away.
- Watery eyes as unshed tears rise to the surface.
- Nasal discharges, sneezing, coughing as suppressed emotion escapes.

■ Throat disorders as the need for self-expression, creativity and change emerges.

■ Initial tiredness after a treatment as the body heals itself.

■ A healing crisis whereby previous illnesses that have been suppressed flare up temporarily and then disappear.

Before you begin your hand reflexology treatment check:

■ You have created the right ambience (see Chapter 3)

■ All jewellery has been removed so as not to scratch the receiver.

■ Your nails are clipped closely and hands are scrupulously clean.

■ You have made the receiver comfortable.

■ You are totally calm and relaxed in body and mind.

■ You have carried out a physical examination of the hands. Remember they reveal a great deal of important information (see page 26).

■ If there any contraindications (see page 27).

Step-by-step sequence: right hand

Relaxation techniques

Warm up the right hand as outlined in Chapter 4. As a memory jogger the relaxation techniques you have mastered are:

1 Greeting the hand.
2 Stroking the hand.
3 Opening the hand.
4 Knuckling the palm.
5 Circling the palm.
6 Loosening the wrist.
7 Moving the wrist.
8 Loosening and moving the fingers and thumbs.
9 Solar plexus release.
10 Stroking the hand with a feather light touch.

Step 1: The Head and Brain

Location: Top, back and sides of the thumb

Rest the receiver's right hand, palm uppermost, on a towel on your pillow/cushion and place your left hand under the receiver's palm. Remember not to grip the receiver's hand too tightly and take tiny little steps. Place the pad of your right thumb on the tip of the receiver's right thumb and walk down several times to the base. Make sure that you cover the outside, back and inside of the thumb. You will probably need to do about 4–6 rows to cover the top, back and sides of the thumb thoroughly.

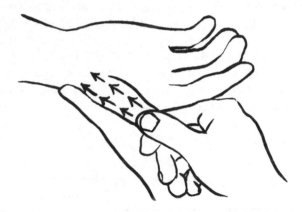

Figure 6.1   Head and brain

Problems which may be alleviated include:

- Headaches
- Migraine
- Poor concentration
- Poor memory
- Parkinson's disease
- Alzheimer's disease
- Stroke
- Multiple sclerosis
- Learning disorders such as dyslexia

- Lack of coordination
- Cerebral palsy
- Attention deficit disorder
- Neuralgia
- Baldness and scalp problems
- After effects of an anaesthetic
- Depression
- Lack of confidence.

Step 2: The Pituitary Gland

Location: Centre of the fleshy part of the back of the thumb

Be prepared to search to pinpoint the pituitary gland. It is often off-centre, slightly higher, lower, to the right or to the left. If you are very lucky, a small lump may be visible or palpable indicating the exact location. With the receiver's hand supported in your left hand, use your right thumb to hook in and back-up over the pituitary gland reflex. It is often a sensitive point.

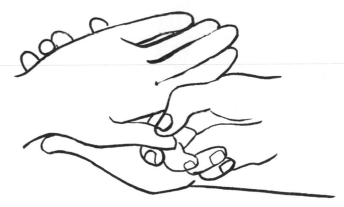

Figure 6.2   Pituitary gland

Problems which may be alleviated include:
- All hormonal imbalances
- Menopause
- Premenstrual syndrome

- Painful, scanty or heavy menstruation
- Endometriosis
- Infertility problems
- Thyroid disorders.

Step 3: The Pineal Gland/Hypothalamus

Location: Just above the pituitary gland

Move your thumb up very slightly towards the tip of the thumb and rock the thumb on to its outer edge to circle over the pineal gland. Then rock your thumb on to its inner edge and use pressure circles to treat the hypothalamus.

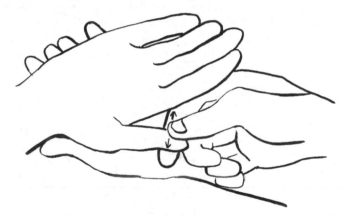

Figure 6.3   Pineal/hypothalamus

Problems which may be alleviated include:

- Seasonal Affective Disorder (SAD)
- Lack of vision
- Lack of intuition
- Hormonal imbalances.

Step 4: The Face

Location: Front of the thumb

Gently turn over the receiver's hand and support it with your left hand. Caterpillar walk down the front of the thumb from the tip of the thumb to its base. You may need to walk down 3–4 times depending on the size of the thumb. If you find it easier you may use your index finger instead.

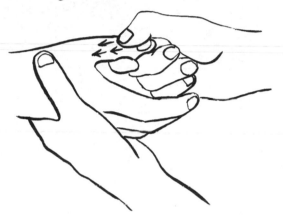

Figure 6.4   The face

Problems which may be alleviated include:

- Eye problems, e.g. conjunctivitis, glaucoma
- Nasal disorders
- Teeth and gum disorders
- Jaw problems
- Facial neuralgia
- Bell's palsy (facial paralysis)
- Facial acne.

Step 5: The Neck

Location: Base of the thumb

Support the receiver's hand with your left hand. Gently hold the receiver's thumb between your index finger and thumb and rotate it both clockwise and anti-clockwise. This is excellent for alleviating a stiff neck. If the thumb grates or does not move very well gently encourage but never force it to move.

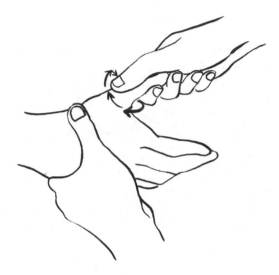

Figure 6.5   Neck rotation

Problems which may be alleviated include:

- Painful neck muscles
- Lack of movement in the neck
- Arthritis in the neck (cervical spondylosis)
- Rheumatoid arthritis
- Whiplash injuries.

Step 6: The Neck/Thyroid/Throat

Location: Back and front of the base of the thumb

Support the receiver's hand, palm uppermost, and use your right thumb to walk across the back of the base of the thumb several times. You will often feel a sensation of grittiness like sandpaper in this area.

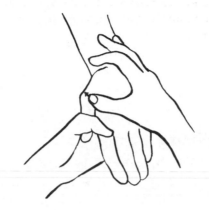

Figure 6.6   Neck/thyroid/throat (back)

Turn the hand over and grasp the thumb between your left thumb and index finger. Use your right thumb to caterpillar walk across the front of the base of the thumb.

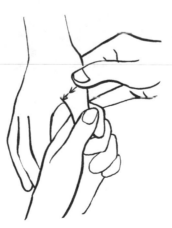

Figure 6.7   Neck/thyroid/throat (front)

Problems which may be alleviatedinclude:

■ All neck problems as outlined in Step 5
■ Throat disorders such as tonsillitis, laryngitis

- Vocal cord problems
- Difficulty in saying what you really think
- Lack of self-expression
- Inability to tell the truth
- Lump in the throat
- Suppressed emotions
- Thyroid and parathyroid disorders.

Step 7: The Sinuses

Location: Top, back and sides of the fingers

Support the receiver's hand, palm uppermost, in the palm of your left hand. Use your right thumb to walk from the tip of the little finger to its base. You will need to do about three rows to cover the area thoroughly. Repeat on the ring, middle and index fingers.

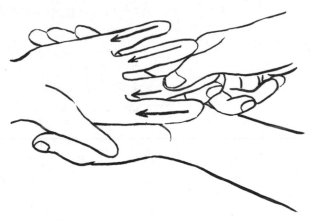

Figure 6.8   Sinuses

To treat the sides of the fingers, you may use your thumb and index finger to walk down both sides at the same time.

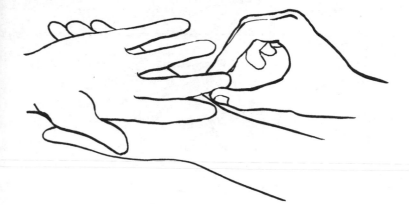

Figure 6.9   Sinuses

Problems which may be alleviated include:
- Sinus problems
- Catarrh
- Allergies
- Hay fever
- Colds
- Loss of sense of smell
- Nasal polyps
- Rhinitis
- Ear problems
- Eye problems.

Step 8: The Teeth

Location: Dorsal side (top) of the fingers

Turn the hand over and support the fingers with your left hand. Commence at the top of the index finger and do about three or four rows of thumb walking to cover the dorsal side of the finger. Repeat on the middle, ring and little fingers.

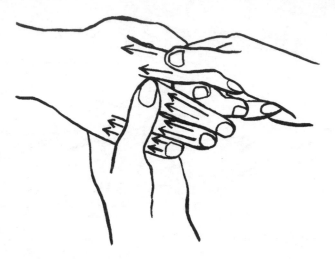

Figure 6.10   Teeth

Problems which may be alleviated include:

- Toothache
- Painful, inflamed or infected gums
- Sensitive teeth
- Tooth abscesses
- Teething.

Step 9: The Upper Lymphatics

Location: Webbing between the fingers

Support with your left hand and using your right thumb and index finger gently squeeze to massage the webbing between each of the fingers.

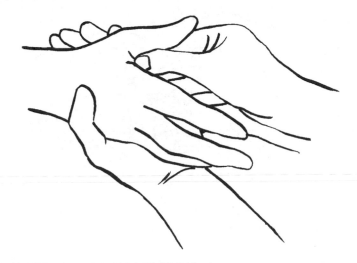

Figure 6.11   Upper lymphatics

Problems which may be alleviated include:

- Toxic lymphatic system caused by poor diet, medications or lack of exercise.
- Infections – especially the ear, nose and throat. This movement will help to drain the head and neck.
- Poor immune function, for instance, where a person suffers from recurrent sinus or throat problems or in cases of ME.

Step 10: The Right Ear/Eustachian Tube/Eye

Location: Along the ridge at the base of the fingers

Support the receiver's right hand, palm uppermost, with your left thumb across their fingers gently holding them back. Use your right thumb to walk across the ridge at the base of the fingers working from the little finger to the index finger.

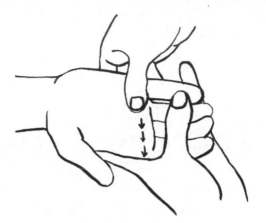

Figure 6.12   General eye/ear area

To pinpoint the right ear, walk slowly across the area again and stop between the fourth and fifth fingers (ring and little finger). Either hook in and back-up or perform pressure circles on the ear point.

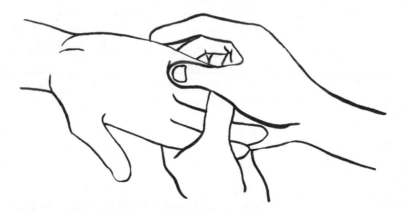

Figure 6.13   Ear

To treat the Eustachian tube take just a few more tiny steps and stop between fingers three and four (middle and ring fingers). Perform pressure circles or hook in and back-up on the Eustachian tube point.

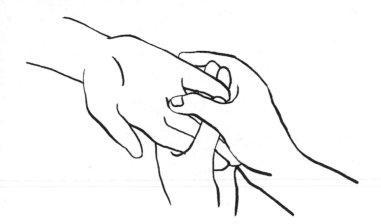

Figure 6.14   Eustachian tube

Continue to walk and stop between fingers two and three (index and middle fingers) to treat the eye point. Either hook in and back-up or use pressure circles to treat the right eye.

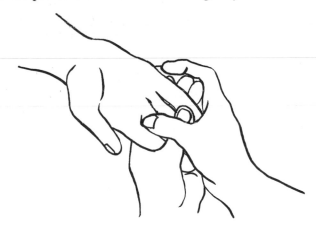

Figure 6.15   Eye

Problems which may be alleviated include:
- Earache
- Ear infections

- Glue ear
- Hearing problems
- Vertigo/dizziness
- Balance problems
- Tinnitus
- Sore eyes
- Watery eyes
- Blocked tear ducts
- Conjunctivitis
- Glaucoma
- Cataracts.

Step 11: The Spine/Sciatic Line

Location: Inner edge of the hand/the wrist

With the receiver's hand, palm uppermost, place your right hand palm down on their hand to steady and support. Place your left thumb on the edge of the hand just below the nail bed and begin to caterpillar walk right down the side of the hand. In your initial steps you are covering the neck area of the spine (cervical vertebrae) continuing down the middle of the back (thoracic vertebrae) and into the lumbar area.

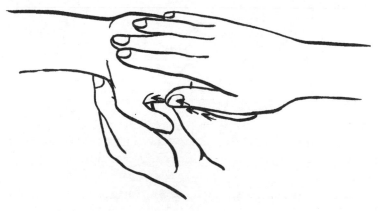

Figure 6.16   Spine

Caterpillar walk right across the wrist with your left thumb in order to treat the sciatic nerve.

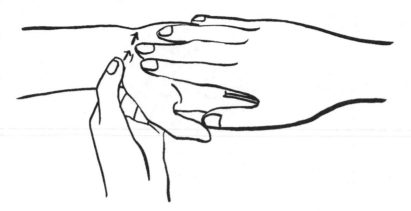

Figure 6.17   Sciatic nerve

You may also use your other thumb to repeat the thumb walking in the opposite direction working across the wrist and then up towards the thumbnail.

Problems which may be alleviated include:
- Backache/neck ache
- Arthritis of the spine
- Disc problems
- Lack of mobility and stiffness in the back
- Sciatica.

Step 12: The Right Lung/Chest Area

Location: Palm of hand from the ridge at the base of the fingers to just above the webbing of the thumb (the diaphragm line)

Clasp the hand, palm uppermost, with your fingers underneath and your thumb gently pressing back the receiver's fingers. Start just below the ridge at the base of the fingers and use your right thumb to caterpillar walk in horizontal strips across the hand. Continue until you reach the diaphragm line.

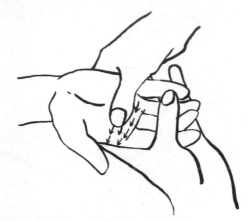

Figure 6.18   Right lung/chest

You may also work on the same area in vertical instead of horizontal strips. Try finger walking with one or more fingers.

Problems which may be alleviated include:

- All lung problems
- Coughs and colds
- Bronchitis
- Emphysema
- Pleurisy
- Asthma
- Hyperventilation
- Panic attacks
- Shallow breathing.

Step 13: The Right Lung/Breast/Mammary Glands

Location: Same area as step 12 but on the dorsum (back) of the hand

Now turn the hand over and rest the receiver's hand on your palm, pressing the fingers gently down with your left thumb. Finger walk in vertical strips down the troughs on top of the hand, from the base of the fingers to the diaphragm line.

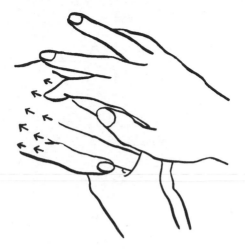

Figure 6.19   Right lung/breast/mammary glands

You may prefer to walk across the hand in horizontal strips.

Problems which may be alleviated include:

- Respiratory problems
- Breast problems such as tenderness due to PMT
- Harmless breast lumps
- Mastitis.

Step 14: The Shoulder

Location: Just below the little finger and above the diaphragm line

Support the receiver's hand and place your right thumb just below the little fingers and use pressure circles to treat the shoulder. This area usually feels very gritty and hard since most people suffer with tension in the shoulders.

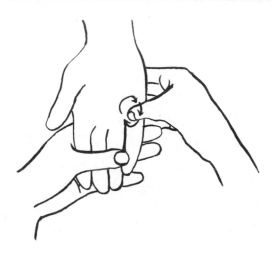

Figure 6.20   Shoulder reflex

Problems which may be alleviated include:
- Tension in the shoulders
- Frozen shoulder
- Arthritis
- Carrying too much responsibility on the shoulders.

Step 15: The Liver/Gallbladder

Location: Right hand only. Zones 3,4,5 between the diaphragm line and the waistline

Support the hand, palm uppermost, with your left thumb over the top of the receiver's fingers to open up the reflex area. Use your right thumb to work from Zone 5, which is the little finger side, to Zone 3.

Pinpoint the gallbladder reflex, which is located roughly in line with the fourth finger. This is often a tender area that may feel like a small indentation or a slight swelling. Use pressure circles to treat this area or the rotation on a point technique by placing the pad of your right thumb on the gallbladder reflex and rotating the hand in a circular motion around the thumb.

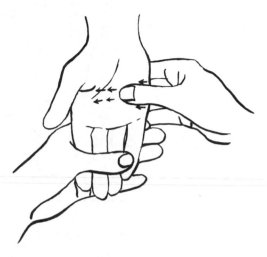

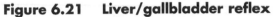

Figure 6.21   Liver/gallbladder reflex

Problems which may be alleviated include:

- Liver problems
- Gallbladder problems
- Nausea
- Difficulties with fat digestion
- Toxicity
- Overindulging in food and/or drink.

Step 16: The Stomach/Pancreas/Duodenum

Location: Zones 1 and 2 between the diaphragm line and the waistline

Using your right hand for support, caterpillar walk with your thumb in horizontal rows from the diaphragm line to the waistline.

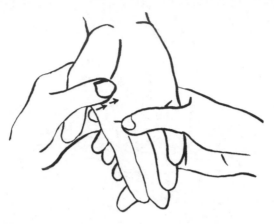

Figure 6.22   Stomach/pancreas/duodenum

Problems which may be alleviated include:
- Indigestion
- Difficulty in digesting food
- Stomach cramps
- Stomach ulcers
- General digestive disorders
- Diabetes
- Low blood sugar (hypoglycaemia).

Step 17: The Right Adrenal Gland

Location: Palm of the hand beneath the index finger just below the webbing of the thumb and index finger

The adrenal glands are easily pinpointed as they are usually tender, since most of us have stress in our lives! Cup the receiver's hand, palm uppermost, with your left hand and use your right thumb to perform pressure circles or press and release over the adrenal reflex. If it is not tender, try the hook in and back-up technique.

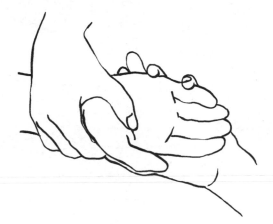

Figure 6.23   Right adrenal gland

Problems which may be alleviated include:

- Stress and tension
- Inflammatory conditions such as rheumatoid arthritis, irritable bowel syndrome
- Allergies
- Lack of energy/exhaustion
- Pain relief.

Step 18: The Right Kidney/Ureter Tube/Bladder

Location: On the waistline between zones 2 and 3

Place the pad of your thumb on the kidney reflex and perform gentle pressure circles. Then caterpillar walk towards Zone 1 on the inside of the hand just above the wrist and use pressure circles to massage the bladder reflex.

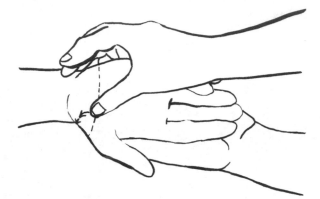

Figure 6.24   Right kidney/ureter/bladder

Problems which may be alleviated include:
- Kidney problems
- Bladder infections such as cystitis
- Bedwetting
- Incontinence
- Fluid retention.

CAUTION

Always work from kidney towards the bladder (*never* bladder to kidney) to avoid transforming a mild bladder infection into a kidney infection, which is obviously more severe.

Step 19: The Small Intestines

Location: Zones 1–4 slightly below the waistline to slightly above the pelvic line

Support the receiver's hand, palm uppermost, with your right hand. Place your left thumb slightly below the waistline on the thumb side of the hand and caterpillar walk in horizontal rows until you are slightly above the pelvic line. You will need to do about three or four rows.

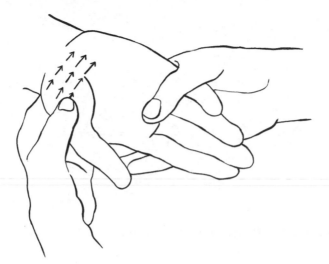

Figure 6.25   Small intestines

Problems which may be alleviated include:
■ All digestive disorders
■ Irritable bowel syndrome
■ Crohn's disease
■ Abdominal bloating
■ Allergies.

Step 20: The Ileocaecal Valve/Appendix/Ascending and Transverse Colons

Location: The colon wraps around the small intestines

The ileocaecal valve and the appendix are located in the right hand only. Place the pad of your right thumb in between Zones 4 and 5 (between the little finger and ring finger) slightly above the wrist. Perform pressure circles, rotation on a point or the hook in and back-up technique on the ileocaecal/appendix reflex. You may feel a small hollow. Walk up towards the waistline (ascending colon) and then turn 90 degrees and walk across the hand just below the waistline until you reach the inside of the hand.

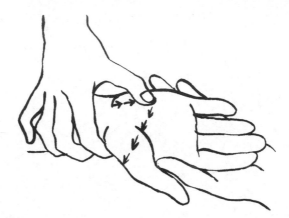

**Figure 6.26   Ileocaecal valve/appendix/ascending/
transverse colons**

You may need to practise this step several times. Adjust your hands
if necessary to make Step 20 as comfortable for your hands as
possible.

Problems which may be alleviated include:
- All digestive problems
- Constipation
- Diarrhoea
- Irritable bowel syndrome
- Crohn's disease
- Ulcerative colitis
- Coeliac disease.

Step 21: The Joints: Right Shoulder, Arm, Elbow, Wrist, Hand, Hip, Leg and Knee

Location: Outer edge of the hand

Hold the receiver's hand, palm uppermost, with your left hand,
thumb on top gently holding the fingers back. Place your right
thumb at the base of the little finger (shoulder joint) and walk down
the outer edge of the hand until you reach the wrist to ensure that
you have covered all the joints thoroughly.

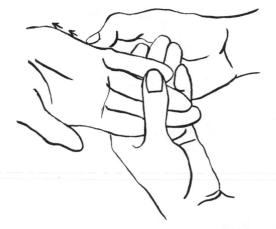

Figure 6.27   Joints: Right shoulder, arm, elbow, wrist, hand, hip, leg and knee

Problems which may be alleviated include:

- All joint problems
- Arthritis
- Frozen shoulder
- Housemaid's knee
- All sports injuries, such as tennis elbow
- Sprains and strains
- Cartilage and ligament problems.

Step 22: The Right Ovary/Testicle

Location: Outer edge (little finger side) of the hand

The reflexes for the reproductive organs are all to be found around the wrist. Grasp the receiver's fingers with your right hand and place the pad of your left thumb on the ovary reflex on the outer edge of the wrist. Use the rotation on a point technique to treat the ovary/testicle.

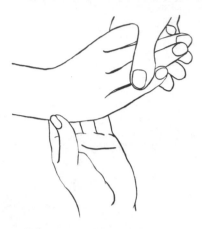

Figure 6.28   Right ovary/testicle

Problems which may be alleviated include:
- All menstrual disorders
- PMT
- Scanty, irregular, heavy menstruation
- Ovarian cysts
- The menopause
- Infertility problems.

CAUTION

If the receiver is pregnant and you are a layperson or a student then omit the reproductive areas (Steps 22, 23 and 24). A fully qualified reflexologist may treat these areas.

Step 23: The Prostate/Uterus

Location: Thumb side of the wrist

Grasp the receiver's fingers with your left hand and place your right thumb on the prostate/uterus reflex. Use the rotation on a point technique.

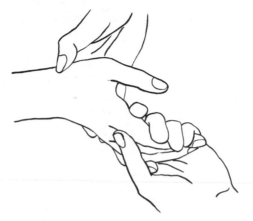

Figure 6.29   Prostate/uterus

Problems which may be alleviated include:
- All menstrual irregularities
- Difficulty in conceiving
- Miscarriage problems
- Prostate problems.

Step 24: The Fallopian Tubes/Vas Deferens/Lymph Nodes of Groin

Location: Circling the wrist

Rest the receiver's hand, palm downwards, on the palm of your hand. Thumb or finger walk right across the wrist on the back of the hand. Then turn the hand over and continue walking across the wrist of the palm of the hand.

Problems which may be alleviated include:
- Problems with the reproductive organs
- Fluid retention
- Toxic accumulation.

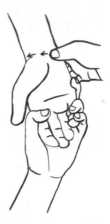

Figure 6.30   Fallopian tube/vas deferens/lymph nodes of groin

Step 25: Completion

Support the receiver's hand and gently stroke both the top and the palm of the hand to ensure that any toxins, which have been released, are dispersed. Sandwich the receiver's hand between both your hands and hold it lightly for about 30 seconds or more to totally relax the receiver.

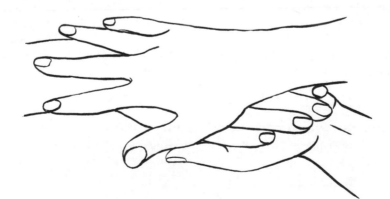

Figure 6.31   Completion

Cover up the right hand

Step-by-step sequences: left hand

Relaxation techniques

Warm up the left hand as outlined in Chapter 4. As a memory jogger the relaxation techniques you have mastered are:

1 Greeting the hand
2 Stroking the hand
3 Opening the hand
4 Knuckling the palm
5 Circling the palm
6 Loosening the wrist
7 Moving the wrist
8 Loosening and moving the fingers and thumbs
9 Solar plexus release
10 Stroking the hand with a feather light touch

Step 1: The Head and Brain

Location: Top, back and sides of the thumb

Rest the receiver's left hand, palm uppermost, on the towel on your pillow/cushion and place your left hand on top of the receiver's palm. Place the pad of your right thumb on the tip of the receiver's left thumb and walk down several times to the base. Remember not to grip the receiver's hand too tightly and take tiny little steps. Make sure that you cover the outside, back and inside of the thumb. You will probably need to do about four to six rows to cover the top, back and sides of the thumb thoroughly.

Problems which may be alleviated include:

■ Headaches
■ Migraine
■ Poor concentration
■ Poor memory
■ Parkinson's disease
■ Alzheimer's disease
■ Stroke
■ Multiple sclerosis

- Learning disorders such as dyslexia
- Lack of coordination
- Cerebral palsy
- Attention deficit disorder
- Neuralgia
- Baldness and scalp problems
- After effects of an anaesthetic
- Depression
- Lack of confidence.

Step 2: The Pituitary Gland

Location: Centre of the fleshy part of the back of the thumb

Be prepared to search to pinpoint the pituitary gland. It is often off-centre, slightly higher, lower, to the right or to the left. If you are very lucky, a small lump may be visible or palpable indicating the exact location. With the palm of your left hand resting on the receiver's palm, use your right thumb to hook in and back-up over the pituitary gland reflex. It is often a sensitive point.

Problems which may be alleviated include:

- All hormonal imbalances
- Menopause
- Premenstrual syndrome
- Painful, scanty or heavy menstruation
- Endometriosis
- Infertility problems
- Thyroid disorders.

Step 3: The Pineal Gland/Hypothalamus

Location: Just above the pituitary gland

Move your thumb up very slightly towards the tip of the thumb and rock the thumb on to its outer edge to circle over the pineal gland. Then rock your thumb on to its inner edge and use pressure circles to treat the hypothalamus.

Problems which may be alleviated include:

- Seasonal Affective Disorder (SAD)
- Lack of vision
- Lack of intuition
- Hormonal imbalances.

Step 4: The Face

Location: Front of the thumb

Gently turn over the receiver's hand and support it with your right hand. With your left thumb caterpillar walk down the front of the thumb from the tip of the thumb to its base. You may need to walk down three or four times depending on the size of the thumb.

Problems which may be alleviated include:

- Eye problems, e.g. conjunctivitis, glaucoma
- Nasal disorders
- Teeth and gum disorders
- Jaw problems
- Facial neuralgia
- Bells palsy (facial paralysis)
- Facial acne.

Step 5: The Neck

Location: Base of the thumb

Support the receiver's hand with your left hand. Gently hold the receiver's thumb between your index finger and thumb and rotate it both clockwise and anti-clockwise. This is excellent for alleviating a stiff neck. If the thumb grates or does not move very well gently encourage it but never force it to move.

Problems which may be alleviated include:

- Painful neck muscles
- Lack of movement in the neck
- Arthritis in the neck (cervical spondylosis)
- Rheumatoid arthritis
- Whiplash injuries.

Step 6: The Neck/Thyroid/Throat

Location: Back and front of the base of the thumb

Stabilize the receiver's hand and use your right thumb to walk across the back of the base of the thumb several times. You will often feel a sensation of grittiness like sandpaper in this area. Turn the receiver's hand over and support it with your right hand. Use your left thumb to caterpillar walk across the front of the base of the thumb.

Problems which may be alleviated include:

- All neck problems as outlined in Step 5
- Throat disorders such as tonsillitis, laryngitis
- Vocal cord problems
- Difficulty in saying what you really think
- Lack of self-expression
- Inability to tell the truth
- Lump in the throat
- Suppressed emotions
- Thyroid and parathyroid disorders.

Step 7: The Sinuses

Location: Top, back and sides of the fingers

Support the receiver's hand, palm uppermost, in the palm of your right hand. Use your left thumb to walk from the tip of the little finger to its base. You will need to do about three rows to cover the area thoroughly. Repeat on the ring, middle and index fingers.

To treat the sides of the fingers, support with your left hand and use your right thumb and index finger to walk down both sides at the same time.

Problems which may be alleviated include:

- Sinus problems
- Catarrh
- Allergies
- Hay fever
- Colds

- Loss of sense of smell
- Nasal polyps
- Rhinitis
- Ear problems
- Eye problems.

Step 8: The Teeth

Location: Dorsal side (top) of the fingers

Turn the hand over and support in a handshake position with your left hand. Commence at the top of the index finger and do several rows of thumb walking to cover the dorsal side of the finger. Repeat on the middle, ring and little fingers.

Problems which may be alleviated include:

- Toothache
- Painful, inflamed or infected gums
- Sensitive teeth
- Tooth abscesses
- Teething.

Step 9: The Upper Lymphatics

Location: Webbing in between the fingers

Support with your left hand and using your right thumb and index finger gently squeeze to massage the webbing between each of the fingers.

Problems which may be alleviated include:

- Toxic lymphatic system caused by poor diet, medications or lack of exercise.
- Infections – especially the ear, nose and throat. This movement will help to drain the head and neck.
- Poor immune function, for instance, where a person suffers from recurrent sinus or throat problems or in cases of ME.

Step 10: The Left Ear/Eustachian Tube/Eye

Location: Along the ridge at the base of the fingers

Support the receiver's left hand, palm uppermost, with your left thumb across their fingers gently holding them back. Use your right thumb to walk across the ridge at the base of the fingers working from the index finger to the little finger.

Walk slowly across the area again and stop between Zones 2 and 3 (index and middle fingers) to treat the eye point. Either hook in and back-up or use pressure circles to treat the right eye.

To treat the Eustachian tube take just a few more tiny steps and stop between Zones 3 and 4 (middle and ring fingers). Perform pressure circles or hook in and back-up on the Eustachian tube point.

Finally, to pinpoint the left ear, stop between the fourth and fifth fingers (ring and little finger). Either hook in and back-up or perform pressure circles on the ear point.

Problems which may be alleviated include:

- Earache
- Ear infections
- Glue ear
- Hearing problems
- Vertigo/dizziness
- Balance problems
- Tinnitus
- Sore eyes
- Watery eyes
- Blocked tear ducts
- Conjunctivitis
- Glaucoma
- Cataracts.

Step 11: The Spine/Sciatic Line

Location: The inner edge of the hand/the wrist

With the receiver's hand palm uppermost, place your left hand palm down on their hand to steady and support. Place your right thumb on the edge of the hand just below the nail bed and begin to caterpillar walk right down the side of the hand. In your initial steps you are covering the neck area of the spine (cervical vertebrae) continuing down the middle of the back (thoracic vertebrae) and into the lumbar area.

Continue to caterpillar walk right across the wrist in order to treat the sciatic nerve.

You may also use your other thumb to repeat the thumb walking in the opposite direction, working across the wrist and then up towards the thumbnail.

Problems which may be alleviated include:

■ Backache/neck ache
■ Arthritis of the spine
■ Disc problems
■ Lack of mobility and stiffness in the back
■ Sciatica.

Step 12: The Left Lung/Chest Area

Location: Palm of hand from the ridge at the base of the fingers to just above the webbing of the thumb (the diaphragm line)

Clasp the hand, palm uppermost with your fingers underneath and your thumb gently pressing back the receiver's fingers. Start just below the ridge at the base of the fingers and use your right thumb to caterpillar walk in horizontal strips across the hand. Continue until you reach the diaphragm line.

You may also work on the same area in vertical instead of horizontal strips. Try finger walking with one or more fingers.

Problems which may be alleviated include:

■ All lung problems
■ Coughs and colds
■ Bronchitis
■ Emphysema
■ Pleurisy
■ Asthma
■ Hyperventilation

■ Panic attacks
■ Shallow breathing.

Step 13: The Heart Area

Location: Left hand only. Zones 2–3 just above the diaphragm line

Support the receiver's hand, palm uppermost, with your left hand and use your right thumb to gently walk across Zones 2 and 3. Also perform several slow pressure circles over the reflex area.

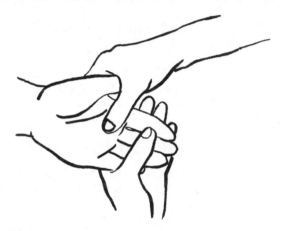

Figure 6.32   Heart area

Problems which may be alleviated include:

■ All heart problems
■ Irregular heat beat
■ High/low blood pressure
■ Circulatory problems
■ Palpitations
■ Inability to love oneself and others
■ Difficulty in displaying affection.

CAUTION

If the receiver feels any pain in the heart area do *not* increase the pressure. If you are not a professional reflexologist it is advisable to omit this area if the receiver has severe heart problems.

Step 14: The Left Lung/Breast/Mammary Glands

Location: Same area as Step 12 but on the dorsum (back) of the hand

Now turn the hand over and rest the receiver's hand on the palm of your left hand. Finger walk in vertical strips down the troughs on top of the hand from the base of the fingers to the diaphragm line.

Problems which may be alleviated include:

- Respiratory problems
- Breast problems such as tenderness due to PMT
- Harmless breast lumps
- Mastitis.

Step 15: The Shoulder

Location: Just below the little finger and above the diaphragm line

Support the receiver's hand and place your left thumb just below the little finger and use pressure circles to treat the shoulder. This area usually feels very gritty and hard since most people suffer with tension in the shoulders.

Problems which may be alleviated include:

- Tension in the shoulders
- Frozen shoulder
- Arthritis
- Carrying too much responsibility on the shoulders.

Step 16: The Spleen

Location: Left hand only. Zones 4–5 between the diaphragm line and the waistline

Support the receiver's left hand with your right hand, fingers underneath and thumb on top. Use your left thumb to caterpillar walk across the hand in horizontal rows from Zone 5 to Zone 4 working between the diaphragm line and the waistline. You will need to do about three to four rows.

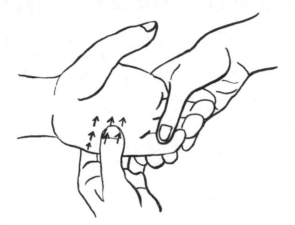

Figure 6.33   Spleen

Problems which may be alleviated include:

■ Poor immune system.

Step 17: The Stomach/Pancreas/Duodenum

Location: Zones 1 and 2 between the diaphragm line and the waistline

Using your left hand for support, caterpillar walk with your right thumb in horizontal rows from the diaphragm line to the waistline.

Problems which may be alleviated include:

■ Indigestion
■ Difficulty in digesting food

- Stomach cramps
- Stomach ulcers
- General digestive disorders
- Diabetes
- Low blood sugar (hypoglycaemia).

Step 18: The Left Adrenal Gland

Location: Palm of the hand beneath the index finger just below the webbing of the thumb and index finger

The adrenal glands are easily pinpointed as they are usually tender, since most of us have stress in our lives! Cup the receiver's hand palm uppermost with your left hand and use your right thumb to perform pressure circles or press and release over the adrenal reflex. If it is not tender, try the hook in and back-up technique.

Problems which may be alleviated include:

- Stress and tension
- Inflammatory conditions such as rheumatoid arthritis, irritable bowel syndrome
- Allergies
- Lack of energy/exhaustion
- Pain relief.

Step 19: The Left Kidney/Ureter Tube/Bladder

Location: On the waistline between Zones 2 and 3

Place the pad of your right thumb on the kidney reflex and perform gentle pressure circles. Then caterpillar walk towards Zone 1 on the inside of the hand just above the wrist and use pressure circles to massage the bladder reflex.

Problems which may be alleviated include:

- Kidney problems
- Bladder infections such as cystitis
- Bedwetting
- Incontinence
- Fluid retention.

CAUTION

Always work from the kidney towards the bladder (*never* bladder to kidney) to avoid transforming a mild bladder infection into a kidney infection, which is more severe.

Step 20: The Small Intestines

Location: Zones 1–4 slightly below the waistline to slightly above the pelvic line

Support the receiver's hand, palm uppermost, with your left hand. Place your right thumb slightly below the waistline on the thumb side of the hand and caterpillar walk in horizontal rows until you are slightly above the pelvic line. You will need to do about three or four rows.

Problems which may be alleviated include:

■ All digestive disorders
■ Irritable bowel syndrome
■ Crohn's disease
■ Abdominal bloating
■ Allergies.

Step 21: The Transverse/Descending Colon/Sigmoid Colon/Rectum

Location: Waistline to pelvic floor line

Support the receiver's hand, palm uppermost, with your left hand. Place your right thumb just below the waistline in Zone 1 and thumb walk across the palm following the waistline until you reach Zone 5. This is the transverse colon. Change hands and caterpillar walk down the hand (descending colon). Just before you reach the wrist, turn your left thumb 90 degrees and walk straight across the palm of the hand (sigmoid colon) to the rectum and anus reflex point.

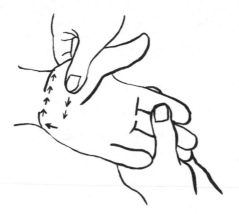

Figure 6.34   Transverse/descending colon/sigmoid colon/rectum

Problems which may be alleviated include:
- All digestive problems
- Constipation
- Diarrhoea
- Irritable bowel syndrome
- Crohn's disease
- Diverticulitis
- Haemorrhoids.

Step 22: The Joints: Left Shoulder, Arm, Elbow, Wrist, Hand, Hip, Leg and Knee

Location: Outer edge of the hand

Hold the receiver's hand, palm uppermost, with your right hand. Place your left thumb at the base of the little finger (shoulder joint) and walk down the outer edge of the hand until you reach the wrist to ensure that you have covered all the joints thoroughly.

Problems which may be alleviated include:
- All joint problems
- Arthritis

■ Frozen shoulder
■ Housemaid's knee
■ All sports injuries, such as tennis elbow
■ Sprains and strains
■ Cartilage and ligament problems.

Step 23: The Left Ovary/Testicle

Location: Outer edge (little finger side) of the wrist

The reflexes for the reproductive organs are all to be found around
the wrist. Grasp the receiver's fingers with your right hand and
place the pad of your left thumb on the ovary reflex on the outer
edge of the wrist. Use the rotation on a point technique to treat the
ovary/testicle.

Problems which may be alleviated include:

■ All menstrual disorders
■ PMT
■ Scanty, irregular, heavy menstruation
■ Ovarian cysts
■ The menopause
■ Infertility problems.

CAUTION

If the receiver is pregnant and you are a layperson or a student,
then omit the reproductive areas (Steps 22, 23 and 24). A fully
qualified reflexologist may treat these areas.

Step 24: The Prostate/Uterus

Location: Thumb side of the wrist

Grasp the receiver's fingers with your left hand and place your
right thumb on the prostate/uterus reflex. Use the rotation on a
point technique.

Problems which may be alleviated include:

- All menstrual irregularities
- Difficulty in conceiving
- Miscarriage problems
- Prostate problems.

Step 25: The Fallopian Tubes/Vas Deferens/Lymph Nodes of Groin

Location: Circling the wrist

Rest the receiver's hand, palm downwards, on the palm of your hand. Thumb or finger walk right across the wrist on the back of the hand. Now turn the hand over and continue walking across the wrist of the palm of the hand.

Problems which may be alleviated include:

- Problems with the reproductive organs
- Fluid retention
- Toxic accumulation.

Step 26: Completion

Support the receiver's hand and gently stroke both the top and the palm of the hand to ensure that any toxins, which have been released, are dispersed. Sandwich the receiver's hand between both your hands and hold it lightly for about 30 seconds or more to totally relax the receiver.

To complete the hand reflexology treatment

1 Return to any reflex areas that were tender during the treatment.
2 Perform several of your favourite relaxation techniques.
3 Massage the hands with your favourite aromatherapy blend to enhance your reflexology treatment (see Chapter 8 for suggestions).
4 With the receiver's hands, palms uppermost, rest the palms of your hands on the receiver's hands. Keep

them there for about a minute visualizing healing energy revitalizing and rejuvenating their whole being. Gradually take away your hands.

5 Allow them to rest for as long as necessary. Offer them a glass of water to flush away any toxins that have been released during the treatment. Advise them to drink plenty of water over the next 24 hours to assist the process of detoxification.

7 | STEP-BY-STEP SELF-TREATMENT

Hand reflexology offers all the benefits of foot reflexology with a big advantage! Hand reflexology is the ideal therapy for self-treatment. It is impossible to perform a complete foot reflexology treatment on oneself, as many of the reflex points are too difficult to reach. However, *all* the reflexology points on the hands can be contacted with ease.

Another advantage of hand reflexology is that you can treat yourself successfully at any time and in any place. On your way to work, on a bus or train, at your place of work during a tea or lunch break, waiting in a long queue to pay for some shopping, sitting at the doctor's or dentist's or when you are relaxing at home watching television. No one need even know what you are doing!

So there are absolutely no excuses why you should not treat yourself at least once a week. If you have an acute problem, such as hay fever, earache, headache, etc. then the unbalanced reflexes may be treated several times daily.

If you are a professional reflexologist, encourage your patients to work on their own hands in between treatments. This will reinforce the reflexology that you are doing and will speed up your patients' recovery time.

The simple routine detailed below is an excellent way of improving and maintaining good health. It is wonderful for de-stressing yourself at the end of a long hard day. Before you start, make yourself as comfortable as possible. Relax in your favourite chair or sit on the sofa. Place a cushion or a pillow on your lap with a towel on top, rest your hand gently on it and you are ready to begin self-treatment. It could not be easier!

The sequence below will probably take 10–15 minutes. It may take longer at first, but you will soon become familiar with the movements and reflex points. If you have been treating others with hand reflexology you will have no trouble at all mastering this routine.

Left hand

Step 1: The Head and Brain

Location: Top, back and sides of the thumb

Starting at the very tip use your right thumb to walk down the back and sides of your left thumb.

Main uses

Headaches, difficulty in concentrating, fatigue, poor memory.

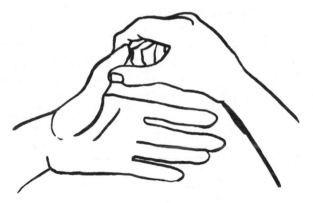

Figure 7.1   Head/brain

Step 2: The Face

Location: Front of the thumb

Use your right thumb, index or middle finger to walk in rows down the front of the thumb.

Main uses

Neuralgia, facial acne, Bell's palsy (facial paralysis), eye, ear, nose, mouth, gum, tooth or jaw problems.

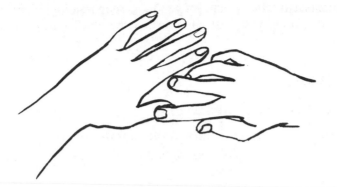

Figure 7.2   Face

Step 3: The Pituitary Gland

Location: Centre of the thumb

Pinpoint the pituitary gland roughly in the centre of the fleshy part of the thumb. You may have to search for it, as it is often slightly off centre – to the left, right, higher or lower. Use the tip of your right thumb either to press and release or hook in and back-up on the pituitary gland.

Main uses

Hormonal problems.

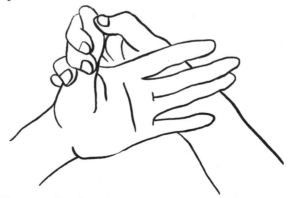

Figure 7.3   Pituitary gland

Step 4: The Pineal Gland/Hypothalamus

Location: Slightly above the pituitary gland

Move your right thumb slightly higher and rock it gently from side to side.

Main uses

SAD (Seasonal Affective Disorder), hormonal imbalances.

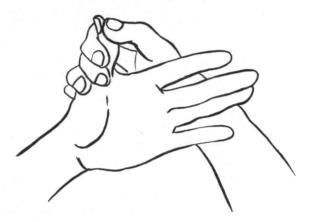

Figure 7.4   Pineal gland/hypothalamus

Step 5: The Neck/Throat/Thyroid

Location: Base of the thumb

First, hold the thumb between your right thumb and index finger, then gently rotate it clockwise and anti-clockwise which is the equivalent of rotating your neck.

Now use your right thumb to walk across both the back and front of the thumb.

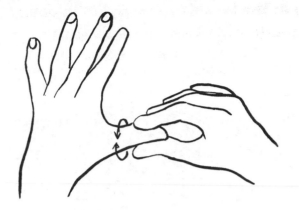

Figure 7.5   Neck rotation

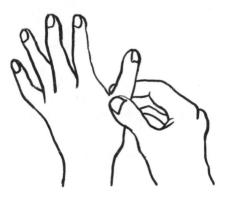

Figure 7.6   Neck/throat/thyroid

Main uses

Neck disorders, tonsillitis, vocal cord problems, thyroid and parathyroid problems.

Step 6: The Sinuses

Location: Back, sides and top of the fingers

Use your thumb and index finger working together to walk down the sides of each finger.

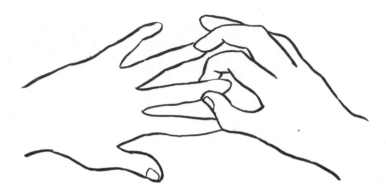

Figure 7.7   Sinuses

If you have sinus problems these movements may be repeated several times as often as required.

Main uses

Sinusitis, hay fever, catarrh, allergies, sinus headaches, nasal polyps.

Step 7: The Teeth

Location: Front of the fingers

Use your right thumb and index finger together to walk down the front and back of each finger. If a tooth is troubling you, you will usually find a tender area on the front of one of the fingers. Gently squeeze your finger and thumb towards each other and hold the pressure for about 30 seconds or until the tenderness subsides.

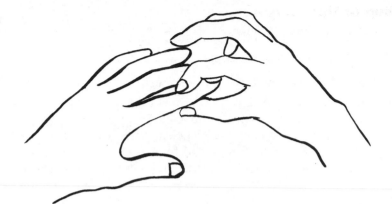

Figure 7.8 Teeth

Main uses
Toothache, abscesses, painful, sensitive or infected gums.

Step 8: The Upper Lymphatics
Location: Webbing between the fingers
With your right thumb and index finger gently squeeze the webbing between each of the fingers.

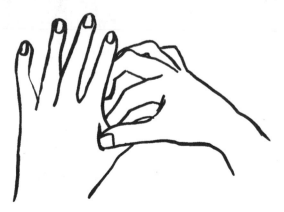

Figure 7.9 Upper lymphatics

Main uses

To build up the body's defences, to drain the head and neck.

Step 9: The Ears and Eyes

Location: Ridge at the base of the fingers

Starting under the little finger walk across the ridge at the base of the fingers. Stop between the fourth and fifth fingers and press and release or hook in and back-up on the ear point. Continue to walk stopping between fingers three and four to treat the Eustachian tube. Finally stop between the middle and index finger to treat the eye point. If you feel any tenderness or crystals perform some pressure circles to clear the reflex.

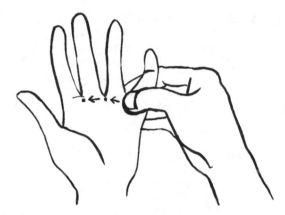

Figure 7.10   Ear/Eustachian tube/eye

Main uses

Earache, hearing problems, vertigo, tinnitus, eye problems such as conjunctivitis, glaucoma and sore or watery eyes. Press the eye point when your eyes feel tired after reading or working at the computer for too long.

Step 10: The Spine

Location: Inside edge (thumb side) of the hand

Place the pad of your right thumb at the base of the left thumbnail on the inner edge of your hand. Caterpillar walk down the inside of the hand until you reach the wrist. You are working the neck (cervical area), mid-back (thoracic area) and lower back (lumbar area).

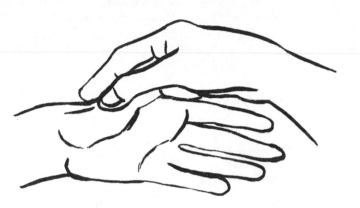

Figure 7.11   Spine

Main uses

Backache, neck ache, lack of mobility, arthritis, disc problems.

Step 11: The Left Lung/Chest

Location: Upper third of the palm of the hand above diaphragm line

With your right thumb caterpillar walk from Zone 5 right across the hand in horizontal rows until you reach the diaphragm line. You will need to do three to four rows.

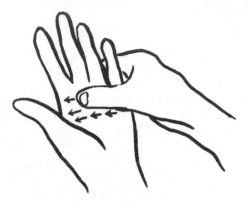

Figure 7.12   Left lung/chest

Main uses

Coughs and colds, asthma, bronchitis, panic attacks.

Step 12: The Solar Plexus

Location: Roughly in the middle of the diaphragm line

Caterpillar walk along the diaphragm line, stop in the centre and perform several pressure circles over the solar plexus.

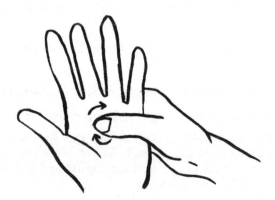

Figure 7.13   Solar plexus

Main uses

Stress and tension.

Step 13: The Left Lung/Breast/Mammary Glands

Location: Upper third of the top of the hand

Turn your hand over and use your index and middle finger or even three fingers to walk down the upper third of the top of the hand starting at the base of the fingers.

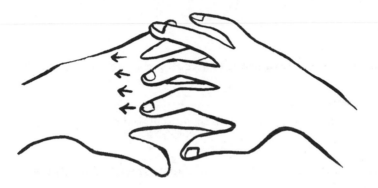

Figure 7.14   Left lung/breast/mammary glands

Main uses

All respiratory problems, breast disorders such as tenderness due to PMT and mastitis.

Step 14: The Stomach/Pancreas/Duodenum/Spleen

Location: Between diaphragm line and waistline

With your palm uppermost, caterpillar walk across in horizontal rows from Zone 5 towards Zone 1. As you walk over Zones 4 and 5 you are treating the spleen (left hand only) and in Zones 1–3 the stomach, pancreas and duodenum.

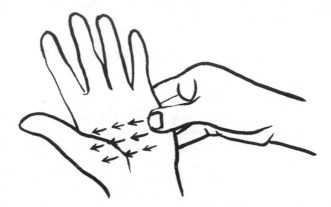

Figure 7.15   Stomach/pancreas/duodenum/spleen

Main uses

All stomach problems such as indigestion and ulcers, general digestive disorders and poor immune function.

Step 15: The Left Adrenal Gland/Kidney/Ureter Tube/Bladder

Location: Below the webbing of the thumb and index finger continuing diagonally towards Zone 1

Press and release on the adrenal gland reflex. Flatten the thumb and move it slightly lower down to treat the kidney reflex with several gentle pressure circles. Walk diagonally towards the inside of the hand to locate the bladder. Perform pressure circles.

Main uses

Stress, pain relief, bladder infections, fluid retention.

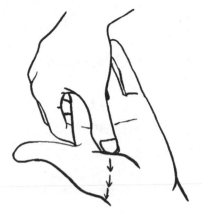

Figure 7.16   Left adrenal gland/kidney/ureter tube/bladder

Step 16: The Small Intestines

Location: Waistline to pelvic floor line Zones 1–4

Caterpillar walk across the lower third of the hand from Zone 4 to Zone 1 of the hand using three to four horizontal rows.

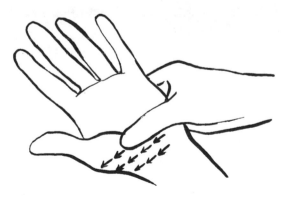

Figure 7.17   Small intestines

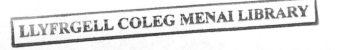

Main uses

All digestive problems.

Step 17: The Transverse/Descending/Sigmoid Colon and Rectum

Location: Lower third of the hand

Place your right thumb just below the waistline in Zone 1 and caterpillar walk across the palm (transverse colon) until you reach Zone 5. Turn your thumb 90 degrees and walk down the hand (descending colon). Just before you reach the wrist turn your thumb 90 degrees and walk straight across the palm of the hand to the rectum and anus.

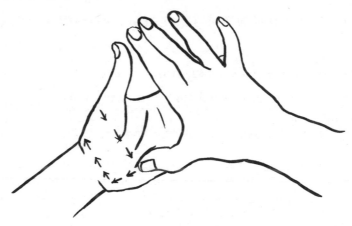

Figure 7.18   Transverse/descending/sigmoid colon/rectum

Main uses

All digestive problems including constipation, diarrhoea, irritable bowel syndrome, diverticulitis, haemorrhoids.

Step 18: The Joints and Sciatic Line

Location: Outer edge of the hand

Place your right thumb at the base of the little finger and walk down the outer edge of the hand until you reach the base of the hand. Walk across the hand just above the wrist to treat the sciatic line.

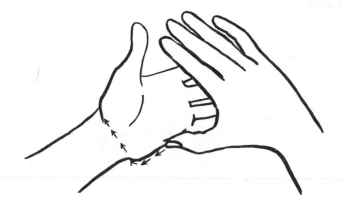

Figure 7.19   Joints and sciatic line

Main uses

All joint problems, sciatica.

Step 19: The Left Ovary/Testicle/Uterus/Prostate

Location: Outer edge (little finger side) and thumb side of the wrist

Place your right thumb on the ovary/testicle point on the outer edge of the wrist. Perform several pressure circles over the area. Now place your index finger on the inside (thumb side) of the wrist to treat the reflex of the uterus/prostate.

Main uses

All menstrual irregularities, difficulty in conceiving, prostate problems.

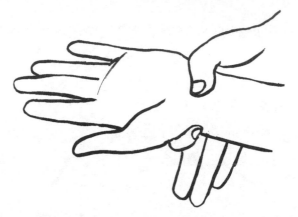

Figure 7.20   Left ovary/testicle/uterus/prostate

Step 20: The Fallopian Tube/Vas Deferens/Lymph Nodes of the Groin

Location: Circles the wrist

Use your right thumb to walk all the way round the wrist both front and back.

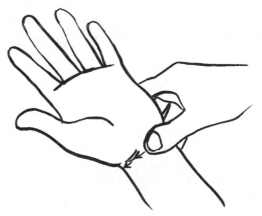

Figure 7.21   Fallopian tube/vas deferens/lymph nodes of groin

Main uses
Toxic accumulation, problems with the reproductive organs, fluid retention.

Right hand

Rest your right hand on a pillow or cushion.

Step 1: The Head and Brain
Location: Top, back and sides of the thumb
Starting at the very tip, use your left thumb to walk down the back and sides of your right thumb.

Main uses
Headaches, difficulty in concentrating, fatigue, poor memory.

Step 2: The Face
Location: Front of the thumb
Use your left thumb, index or middle finger to walk in rows down the front of the thumb.

Main uses
Neuralgia, facial acne, Bell's palsy (facial paralysis), eye, ear, nose, mouth, gum, tooth or jaw problems.

Step 3: The Pituitary Gland
Location: Centre of the thumb
Pinpoint the pituitary gland roughly in the centre of the fleshy part of the thumb. You may have to search for it, as it is often slightly off centre – to the left, right, higher or lower. Use the tip of your left thumb either to press and release or hook in and back-up on the pituitary reflex.

Main uses
Hormonal problems.

Step 4: The Pineal Gland/Hypothalamus

Location: Slightly above the pituitary gland

Move your left thumb slightly higher and rock it gently from side to side.

Main uses

SAD (seasonal affective disorder), hormonal imbalances.

Step 5: The Neck/Throat/Thyroid

Location: Base of the thumb

First, hold the thumb between your left thumb and index finger, then gently rotate it clockwise and anti-clockwise which is the equivalent of rotating your neck.

Now use your left thumb to walk across both the back and front of the thumb.

Main uses

Neck disorders, tonsillitis, vocal cord problems, thyroid and parathyroid problems.

Step 6: The Sinuses

Location: Back, sides and top of the fingers

Use your thumb and index finger working together to walk down the sides of each finger. If you have sinus problems these movements may be repeated several times as often as required.

Main uses

Sinusitis, hay fever, catarrh, allergies, sinus headaches, nasal polyps.

Step 7: The Teeth

Location: Front of the fingers

Use your left thumb and index finger together to walk down the front and back of each finger. If a tooth is troubling you will usually find a tender area on the front of one of the fingers. Gently squeeze your finger and thumb towards each other and hold the pressure for about 30 seconds or until the tenderness subsides.

Main uses

Toothache, abscesses, painful, sensitive or infected gums.

Step 8: The Upper Lymphatics

Location: Webbing between the fingers

With your left thumb and index finger gently squeeze the webbing between each of the fingers.

Main uses

To build up the body's defences, to drain the head and neck.

Step 9: The Ears and Eyes

Location: Ridge at the base of the fingers

Starting under the little finger use your left thumb to walk across the ridge at the base of the fingers. Stop between the fourth and fifth fingers and press and release or hook in and back-up on the ear point. Continue to walk stopping between fingers three and four to treat the Eustachian tube. Finally stop between the middle and index finger to treat the eye point. If you feel any tenderness or crystals perform some pressure circles to clear the reflex.

Main uses

Earache, hearing problems, vertigo, tinnitus, eye problems such as conjunctivitis, glaucoma and sore or watery eyes. Press the eye point when your eyes feel tired after reading or working at the computer for too long.

Step 10: The Spine

Location: Inside edge (thumb side) of the hand

Place the pad of your left thumb at the base of the right thumbnail on the inner edge of your hand. Caterpillar walk down the inside of the hand until you reach the wrist. You are working the neck (cervical area), mid-back (thoracic area) and lower back (lumbar area).

Main uses

Backache, neck ache, lack of mobility, arthritis, disc problems.

Step 11: The Right Lung/Chest

Location: Upper third of the palm of the hand above diaphragm line

With your left thumb caterpillar walk from Zone 5 right across the hand in horizontal rows until you reach the diaphragm line. You will need to do three to four rows.

Main uses

Coughs and colds, asthma, bronchitis, panic attacks.

Step 12: The Solar Plexus

Location: Roughly in the middle of the diaphragm line

Caterpillar walk along the diaphragm line, stop in the centre and perform several pressure circles over the solar plexus.

Main uses

Stress and tension.

Step 13: The Right Lung/Breast/Mammary Glands

Location: Upper third of the top of the hand

Turn your hand over and use your index and middle finger or even three fingers to walk down the upper third of the top of the hand starting at the base of the fingers.

Main uses

All respiratory problems, breast disorders such as tenderness due to PMT and mastitis.

Step 14: The Liver/Gallbladder/Stomach/Pancreas/ Duodenum

Location: Zones 1–5 between the diaphragm line and the waistline

Supporting your hand, palm uppermost, walk from Zone 5 (little finger side) to Zone 1 between the diaphragm line and the waistline. As you work from Zones 5 to 3 you are treating the liver and gallbladder. Zones 1 and 2 are the stomach, pancreas and duodenum. Try to pinpoint the gallbladder reflex roughly in line with the fourth finger and use the press and release technique to treat it.

Main uses

Liver/gallbladder problems, overindulgence in food and/or drink, indigestion, stomach cramps and ulcers.

Step 15: The Right Adrenal Gland/Kidney/Ureter Tube/Bladder

Location: Below the webbing of the thumb and index finger continuing diagonally towards zone one

Press and release on the adrenal gland reflex. Flatten the thumb and move it slightly lower down to treat the kidney reflex with several gentle pressure circles. Walk diagonally towards the inside of the hand to locate the bladder. Perform pressure circles.

Main uses

Stress, pain relief, bladder infections, fluid retention.

Step 16: The Small Intestines

Location: Waistline to pelvic floor line Zones 1–4

Caterpillar walk across the lower third of the hand from Zone 4 to Zone 1 of the hand using three to five horizontal rows.

Main uses

All digestive problems.

Step 17: The Ileocaecal Valve/Appendix/Ascending/ Transverse Colons

Location:

Place your left thumb between Zones 4 and 5 (in between the little finger and ring finger) slightly above the wrist. Press and release to treat the ileocaecal valve and appendix. Caterpillar walk up towards the waistline (ascending colon), turn the thumb 90 degrees to walk across the hand just below the waistline (transverse colon) until you reach the other side of the palm.

Main uses

All digestive disturbances.

Step 18: The Joints and Sciatic Line

Location: Outer edge of the hand

Place your left thumb at the base of the little finger and walk down the outer edge of the hand until you reach the base of the hand. Walk across the hand just above the wrist to treat the sciatic line.

Main uses

All joint problems, sciatica.

Step 19: The Right Ovary/Testicle/Uterus/Prostate

Location: Thumb side and outer edge (little finger side) of wrist

Place your left thumb on the uterus/prostate point on the inner edge of the wrist (thumb side). Perform several pressure circles over the area. Now place your index finger on the outside (little finger side) of the wrist to treat the reflex of the ovary/testicle.

Main uses

All menstrual irregularities, difficulty in conceiving, prostrate problems.

Step 20: The Fallopian Tube/Vas Deferens/Lymph Nodes of the Groin

Location: Circles the wrist

Use your left thumb to walk all the way round the wrist both front and back.

Main uses

Toxic accumulation, problems with the reproductive organs, fluid retention.

8 | ESSENTIAL OILS FOR THE HANDS

This chapter describes how essential oils may be used both to enhance your hand reflexology treatments and to care for your hands. We often forget about looking after our precious hands. People use all sorts of creams and potions on their faces in an attempt to banish wrinkles and some even resort to plastic surgery. However, it is our hands that really reveal our age. We need to protect, nurture and massage them regularly.

Why blend your own oils and creams for the hands? Why not just buy commercially produced products? Unfortunately these ready-made creams and oils contain synthetic substances such as preservatives, dyes and fragrances which can damage the skin and may also promote premature ageing of the skin. Commercial products are not only inferior – they also cost far more than homemade blends. The advertising and packaging costs are high and profit is important to both manufacturer and retailer.

When you create your own blends you know that they are therapeutic, pure, natural, freshly made and carry no risk of side effects. It is also very satisfying and a lot of fun!

Essential oils and hand reflexology

The healing powers of essential oils may be harnessed prior to the reflexology treatment, at the end of the session and between treatments to complement and reinforce the work that you are doing.

Do *not* use them during your step-by-step hand reflexology routine. If you do your hands may become too oily and sticky. This makes it virtually impossible to pinpoint and treat the reflex areas as your hands will slip and slide. It also makes it difficult to palpate the reflex points and become aware of the sensitive areas requiring attention.

Using essential oils prior to a treatment

An aromatherapy hand bath is a wonderful way to enjoy the benefits of essential oils prior to a reflexology session.

Preparing and using your hand bath

Find a small bowl and fill it with hand-hot water. Add six drops in total of your chosen undiluted pure essential oil(s) to the bowl of water. Agitate the water to disperse the essential oils(s) thoroughly. If you desire you may blend your essential oils with a teaspoon of carrier oil. Choose any pure, unrefined, cold-pressed, additive-free vegetable, nut or seed oil and blend your six drops of essential oil with it and then add to the hand bath.

Ask the receiver to immerse his/her hands in the hand bath for a few minutes and dry the hands off thoroughly before you start the treatment.

Aromatherapy hand baths are optional but offer the following benefits. They:

- Create a pleasurable and therapeutic aroma for both you and the receiver
- Relax the receiver
- Reduce swelling in the hands
- Alleviate pain and stiffness
- Relieve itching and irritation
- Help cracked and chapped skin
- Complement the treatment in helping to alleviate specific health problems.

Using essential oils at the end of a treatment

As a wonderful dessert, and to reinforce the work you have done, massage the hands thoroughly with your specially blended creams and oils tailor-made for the individual.

Preparing an oil blend

Essential oils are highly concentrated in their pure state and must be blended with a carrier oil. This vegetable, nut or seed oil must be cold pressed, unrefined and additive-free. Mineral oil, such as commercial baby oil, is not really suitable since it tends to clog the pores and prevents the skin from breathing. Sweet almond, apricot kernel and peach kernel are particularly recommended since they are suitable for all skin types, are not too heavy or thick to work with and do not have a strong odour.

A teaspoon holds about 5 ml of carrier oil. If you blend 10 ml (2 teaspoons) there should be plenty left over for the receiver to use between treatments. For your treatment blend just add 3 drops of essential oil to 10 ml (2 teaspoons) of carrier oil.

If you wish to make up a larger quantity for daily use between treatments, then you will need to store your blend in an amber glass bottle since essential oils are damaged by ultra-violet light. A blend will keep for about three to six months if it is stored in an amber coloured bottle away from sunlight. The appropriate dilutions are as follows: -

- 3 drops of essential oil to 10 ml (2 teaspoons) of carrier oil
- 6 drops of essential oil to 20 ml of carrier oil
- 15 drops of essential oil to 50 ml of carrier oil
- 30 drops of essential oil to 100 ml of carrier oil.

Preparing a hand cream

When adding essential oils to a cream base ensure that the cream is non-mineral, lanolin-free and preferably organic for optimum results. Aromatherapy suppliers usually produce suitable creams (see Useful Addresses). You will need amber glass jars to store your creams to preserve their therapeutic properties. The 30 g and 60 g amber coloured jars are the most appropriate for your use.

Choosing your oils for the systems

Essential oil blends can greatly improve the majority of conditions. I have included several recipes for each of the systems of the body.

Circulation

To boost circulation

Essential oil blends and creams are an excellent way of stimulating the circulation, particularly when coupled with massage.

Essential oils include: black pepper, geranium, ginger, lemon, marjoram and rosemary.

Suggested formula:

1 drop of black pepper	in 10 ml of carrier oil
1 drop of geranium	or
1 drop of ginger	10 g of cream
2 drops of black pepper	
2 drops of geranium	Hand bath
2 drops of ginger	

To decrease blood pressure

Useful essential oils include: chamomile, clary sage, frankincense, geranium, lavender, marjoram, neroli, rose and ylang ylang.

Suggested formula:

1 drop of chamomile	in 10 ml of carrier oil
1 drop of geranium	or
1 drop of lavender	10 g of cream
2 drops of chamomile	
2 drops of geranium	Hand bath
2 drops of lavender	

To boost the immune system

Effective essential oils include: bergamot, chamomile, lavender, lemon, tea tree and thyme.

Suggested formula:

1 drop of bergamot	in 10 ml of carrier oil
1 drop of chamomile	or
1 drop of tea tree	10 g of cream
2 drops of bergamot	
2 drops of chamomile	Hand bath
2 drops of tea tree	

Digestion

Constipation

Recommended essential oils include: black pepper, ginger, juniper, marjoram, rose, and rosemary.

Suggested formula:

1 drop of black pepper	in 10 ml of carrier oil
1 drop of juniper	or
1 drop of marjoram	10 g of cream
2 drops of black pepper	
2 drops of juniper	Hand bath
2 drops of marjoram	

Irritable bowel syndrome

Useful essential oils include: chamomile, geranium, ginger, lavender, mandarin, neroli, patchouli, peppermint and rosemary.

Suggested formula:

1 drop of chamomile	in 10 ml of carrier oil
1 drop of geranium	or
1 drop of mandarin	10 g of cream
2 drops of chamomile	
2 drops of geranium	Hand bath
2 drops of mandarin	

Heartburn/Indigestion

Invaluable essential oils include: basil, bergamot, black pepper, cardamon, carrot seed, dill, ginger, lemon, peppermint, rosemary and spearmint.

Suggested formula:

1 drop of carrot seed	in 10 ml of carrier oil
1 drop of ginger	or
1 drop of lemon	10 g of cream
2 drops of carrot seed	
2 drops of ginger	Hand bath
2 drops of lemon	

Emotions/Nerves

Stress

Effective essential oils include: benzoin, bergamot, cedarwood, chamomile, clary sage, frankincense, geranium, jasmine, lavender, mandarin, marjoram, neroli, patchouli, rose, sandalwood, ylang ylang.

Suggested formula:

1 drop of bergamot	in 10 ml of carrier oil
1 drop of frankincense	or
1 drop of sandalwood	10 g of cream
2 drops of bergamot	
2 drops of frankincense	Hand bath
2 drops of sandalwood	

Depression

Uplifting essential oils include: benzoin, bergamot, clary sage, frankincense, geranium, grapefruit, jasmine, lavender, mandarin, marjoram, neroli, rose, rosewood, sandalwood and ylang ylang.

Suggested formula:

1 drop of geranium	in 10 ml of carrier oil
1 drop of grapefruit	or
1 drop of rosewood	10 g of cream
2 drops of geranium	
2 drops of grapefruit	Hand bath
2 drops of rosewood	

Insomnia

Sleep-inducing essential oils include: chamomile, clary sage, lavender, marjoram, neroli and sandalwood.

Suggested formula:

1 drop of chamomile	in 10 ml of carrier oil
1 drop of lavender	or
1 drop of marjoram	10 g of cream
2 drops of chamomile	
2 drops of lavender	Hand bath
2 drops of marjoram	

Kidneys and Bladder

Cystitis

Recommended essential oils include: bergamot, cajeput, frankincense, juniper, lavender, myrtle, sandalwood, tea tree and thyme.

Suggested formula:

1 drop of bergamot	in 10 ml of carrier oil
1 drop of frankincense	or
1 drop of tea tree	10 g of cream
2 drops of bergamot	
2 drops of frankincense	Hand bath
2 drops of tea tree	

Prostate problems

Useful essential oils include: chamomile, cypress, juniper, lavender, sandalwood and tea tree.

Suggested formula:

1 drop of cypress	in 10 ml of carrier oil
1 drop of juniper	or
1 drop of sandalwood	10 g of cream
2 drops of cypress	
2 drops of juniper	Hand bath
2 drops of sandalwood	

Libido

Male formula

Effective essential oils include: cardamon, cinnamon, coriander, ginger, jasmine, patchouli, rose, rosewood, sandalwood and ylang ylang.

Suggested formula:

1 drop of cardamon	in 10 ml of carrier oil
1 drop of rosewood	or
1 drop of ylang ylang	10 g of cream
2 drops of cardamon	
2 drops of rosewood	Hand bath
2 drops of ylang ylang	

Female formula

Sensual essential oils include: clary sage, geranium, jasmine, neroli, patchouli, rose, sandalwood and ylang ylang.

Suggested formula:

1 drop of jasmine	in 10 ml of carrier oil
1 drop of neroli	or
1 drop of rose	10 g of cream
2 drops of jasmine	
2 drops of neroli	Hand bath
2 drops of rose	

Menstrual Cycle

PMT

Invaluable essential oils include: bergamot, chamomile, clary sage, cypress, geranium, grapefruit, jasmine, neroli, rose, sandalwood and ylang ylang.

Suggested formula:

1 drop of bergamot	in 10 ml of carrier oil
1 drop of clary sage	or
1 drop of jasmine	10 g of cream
2 drops of bergamot	
2 drops of clary sage	Hand bath
2 drops of jasmine	

Menopause

Effective essential oils include: chamomile, cypress, geranium, jasmine, juniper, neroli, rose and yarrow.

Suggested formula:

1 drop of chamomile	in 10 ml of carrier oil
1 drop of cypress	or
1 drop of rose	10 g of cream
2 drops of chamomile	
2 drops of cypress	Hand bath
2 drops of rose	

Muscles and Joints

Arthritis

Excellent essential oils include: black pepper, cajeput, chamomile, frankincense, ginger, juniper, lemon, marjoram, myrrh and rosemary.

Suggested formula:

1 drop of chamomile	in 10 ml of carrier oil
1 drop of juniper	or
1 drop of lavender	10 g of cream

2 drops of chamomile
2 drops of juniper   Hand bath
2 drops of lavender

Aches and Pains

Pain relieving essential oils include: cajeput, chamomile, eucalyptus, ginger, lavender, marjoram, peppermint and rosemary.

Suggested formula:

1 drop of chamomile   in 10 ml of carrier oil
1 drop of marjoram   or
1 drop of peppermint   10 g of cream

2 drops of chamomile
2 drops of marjoram   Hand bath
2 drops of peppermint

Respiratory System

Asthma

Effective essential oils include: basil, benzoin, frankincense, lavender and myrrh.

Suggested formula:

1 drop of frankincense   in 10 ml of carrier oil
1 drop of lavender   or
1 drop of myrrh   10 g of cream

2 drops of frankincense
2 drops of lavender   Hand bath
2 drops of myrrh

Coughs and Colds

Recommended essential oils include: benzoin, cajeput, eucalyptus, frankincense, ginger, lemon and rosemary.

Suggested formula:

1 drop of benzoin   in 10 ml of carrier oil
1 drop of cajeput   or
1 drop of ginger   10 g of cream

2 drops of benzoin
2 drops of cajeput   Hand bath
2 drops of ginger

Sinusitis

Decongestive essential oils include: basil, cajeput, eucalyptus, lavender, lemon and tea tree.

Suggested formula:

1 drop of cajeput   in 10 ml of carrier oil
1 drop of lavender   or
1 drop of lemon   10 g of cream

2 drops of cajeput
2 drops of lavender   Hand bath
2 drops of lemon

Skin

Dry, cracked, chapped

Nourishing essential oils include: benzoin, carrot seed, chamomile, frankincense, geranium, jasmine, myrrh, neroli, palmarosa, patchouli and rose.

Suggested formula:

1 drop of benzoin   in 10 ml of carrier oil
1 drop of myrrh   or
1 drop of patchouli   10 g of cream

2 drops of benzoin
2 drops of myrrh   Hand bath
2 drops of patchouli

Mature

Anti-ageing essential oils include: carrot seed, clary sage, frankincense, geranium, jasmine, lavender, neroli, palmarosa, rose and yarrow.

Suggested formula:

1 drop of frankincense   in 10 ml of carrier oil
1 drop of geranium   or
1 drop of neroli   10 g of cream

2 drops of frankincense
2 drops of geranium   Hand bath
2 drops of neroli

Allergies

Invaluable essential oils include: benzoin, chamomile, geranium, lavender, myrrh, patchouli, sandalwood and yarrow.

Suggested formula:

1 drop of chamomile   in 10 ml of carrier oil
1 drop of lavender   or
1 drop of yarrow   10 g of cream

2 drops of chamomile
2 drops of lavender   Hand bath
2 drops of yarrow

Hand exercises

It is essential to exercise your hands regularly to keep them supple, increase strength and heighten sensitivity. Below are some useful exercises.

1 Hold a small ball in your hand and squeeze and relax your fingers around the ball repeatedly. Exercise your other hand in the same way. This exercise will increase strength and flexibility.

2 Gently pull and stretch out the thumb and fingers of each hand one by one. Then circle them clockwise and anticlockwise. This will help to keep finger joints supple and improve mobility.

3 Throw out your fingers so that they are separated and extended as far as possible to improve flexibility.

4 With fingers relaxed, circle both wrists clockwise and anti-clockwise. You can also perform this movement with your fists clenched. This exercise keeps the wrists flexible and also helps to reduce any puffiness.

5 Shake your hands out from the wrists as loosely and rapidly as possible. This will help to relieve both physical and mental tension.

6 Place the palms of your hands in a prayer position. Rub your hands together rapidly. Notice the heat produced by this movement and how wonderful you feel.

7 Place the palms of your hands close to each other so that they are almost touching. Close your eyes and feel any unusual sensations such as tingling, heat or vibrations. Now slowly separate your hands so that they are about 5 cm (2″) apart. Return them to their original position. Expand the gap to about 15 cm (6″) becoming aware of any sensations. This exercise will help to increase your sensitivity – the more you practise the more you will feel.

9 HAND REFLEXOLOGY FOR COMMON AILMENTS: AN A–Z

In this chapter some of the most common conditions will be outlined briefly together with the reflex points on the hands, which can provide relief. If problems persist or are serious you should consult your doctor. Remember, reflexology is an excellent way to support conventional treatment.

Acne

Brief description

It occurs primarily during puberty but may affect adults. Acne is caused by overactivity of the sebaceous glands (oil secreting glands) of the skin. Excess of sebum causes proliferation of bacteria and the pores become blocked, resulting in blackheads, spots and even scarring.

Areas to treat

- Face
- Adrenal glands
- Solar plexus
- Pituitary gland
- All lymph glands
- Large and small intestines
- Liver
- Kidneys
- Lungs
- Thyroid/parathyroids
- Ovaries/testes
- Uterus/prostate.

Allergies

Brief description

The body's immune system overreacts to certain foods, preservatives, tree and flower pollen, dust, animal hair, medications, chemicals and various other substances. It perceives these substances as foreign and therefore displays a defensive reaction. Symptoms include itching, wheals, red patches and swelling of the mucous membranes.

Areas to treat

- Adrenal glands
- Pituitary gland
- Solar plexus
- Diaphragm
- Lungs
- All lymph glands
- Ears
- Eyes
- Eustachian tube
- Nose
- Throat
- Large and small intestines, stomach, liver, gallbladder.

Anaemia

Brief description

The most common disorder caused by a deficiency of the haemoglobin (iron containing) component of the red blood cells. Main symptoms include fatigue, tendency to tire easily, dizziness, palpitations, rapid pulse, loss of appetite and pallor of the skin. It can be caused by loss of blood, as in menstruation, or bleeding from the gastrointestinal tract, in pregnancy and by poor diet.

Areas to treat

- Spleen
- Adrenals

- Heart
- Solar plexus
- Pituitary gland
- Large and small intestines.

Arthritis (osteoarthritis and rheumatoid arthritis)

Brief description

Osteoarthritis is a common degenerative disorder of the joints affecting most people over the age of 60 to some degree. The most commonly affected joints are the weight-bearing joints (hips and knees). Cartilage is destroyed exposing the underlying bone and symptoms include pain, stiffness (especially in the mornings) and limitation of movement.

Rheumatoid arthritis is a chronic inflammatory condition that may affect the whole body although the joints most commonly involved are the hands, wrists, feet and ankles. The affected joints are swollen, painful and stiff and may become deformed. Rheumatoid arthritis is more prevalent in women but the cause is unknown.

Areas to treat

- Adrenal glands
- Solar plexus
- Pituitary gland
- Spine
- Kidneys
- Large and small intestines
- Joints
- Lymphatics.

Asthma

Brief description

It is characterized by wheezing and difficulty in breathing. This is due to narrowing of the bronchial tubes reducing airflow in and out of the lungs. External causes can be irritants or allergens such as pollen, house dust, fur, foods and pollutants as well as stress and anxiety.

Areas to treat
- Lungs
- Diaphragm
- Solar plexus
- Adrenals
- Spine
- Heart
- Lymphatics.

Back problems

Brief description

The spine comprises seven cervical vertebrae, 12 thoracic vertebrae, five lumbar, the sacrum and the coccyx. All of these areas can cause problems such as sciatica, disc problems, limitation of movement and general aches and pains. The majority of us suffer with backache at some time in our lives.

Areas to treat
- Spine (cervical, thoracic and lumbar)
- Sciatic nerve
- Joints
- Adrenals
- Solar plexus
- Diaphragm.

Massage is a powerful tool for alleviating aches and pains. Essential oils are also a powerful method of providing pain relief (see *Teach Yourself Massage* and *Teach Yourself Aromatherapy* by the same author).

Bladder problems (cystitis, incontinence, etc.)

Brief description

The most common bladder problems are infections, such as cystitis, and incontinence particularly after having had children. Typical symptoms include burning sensations while passing water, frequent urination, low backache, abdominal pains, aching in the groin, urination when coughing or laughing.

Areas to treat
- Bladder
- Kidneys
- Ureters
- Lower spine
- Adrenals
- Solar plexus
- Lymphatics.

Bronchitis

Brief description

An inflammatory disease of the respiratory system. Bacteria, viruses, colds or irritants, such as smoke or chemicals, may cause it. The main symptoms are fever, cough and greenish-yellow mucus which may contain blood.

Areas to treat
- Lungs
- Diaphragm
- Lymphatics
- Spine
- Ears
- Eyes
- Nose
- Solar plexus

■ Adrenal glands
■ Heart
■ Large and small intestines

Colds/coughs

Brief description

Sore throat, sneezing, watery eyes, coughing, swollen lymph glands, feeling generally unwell, fever and tiredness are some of the many symptoms of the common cold. It is caused by exposure to bacteria and viruses.

Areas to treat

■ Lungs
■ Nose
■ Throat
■ Ears
■ Eyes
■ Lymphatics
■ Sinuses
■ Solar plexus
■ Diaphragm
■ Adrenals.

Constipation

Brief description

This extremely widespread complaint is caused by poor diet (in particular lack of fibre), inadequate intake of water, lack of exercise, stress, regular use of laxatives and certain drugs such as painkillers, which may make the bowel lazy.

Areas to treat

■ Large and small intestines
■ Ileocaecal valve
■ Anus

- Liver/Gallbladder
- Stomach/Pancreas/Duodenum
- Solar plexus
- Adrenals
- Diaphragm
- Spine.

Massage of the abdomen is also excellent for constipation (see *Teach Yourself Massage* by the same author for details).

Depression

Brief description

A prevalent condition evidenced by the number of prescriptions for antidepressants. Sufferers experience negative emotions, which affects their ability to function. There are many forms of depression ranging from mild temporary depression to very severe cases where suicide may be attempted.

Areas to treat

- Head and brain
- Solar plexus
- Heart
- Pituitary gland
- Lungs
- Diaphragm
- Adrenals
- Pineal.

Ear problems

Brief description

Symptoms may include: fever, pain, secretion from the ear if there is an infection, impaired hearing or even loss of hearing, dizziness or constant noise in the ears (tinnitus).

Areas to treat

- Ear
- Eustachian tube
- Neck
- Sinuses
- Lymphatics – especially upper
- Throat
- Adrenals
- Solar plexus.

Eye disorders

Brief description

There are many eye problems that may be treated with hand reflexology. These include impaired vision, long and shortsightedness, conjunctivitis, watery or tired eyes, squints, glaucoma, burning eyes, blocked tear ducts, feelings of pressure behind the eyes and headaches.

Areas to treat

- Eyes
- Neck
- Cervical spine
- Head and brain
- Solar plexus
- Adrenals.

Flatulence

Brief description

Flatulence is caused by an excessive accumulation of gases in the intestines. It is characterized by a feeling of bloatedness after meals, abdominal cramps and unpleasant smelling gas emissions from the anus. Flatulence may be caused by a poor diet, certain foods and not chewing food properly.

Areas to treat

- Large and small intestines
- Stomach/pancreas/duodenum
- Spine
- Solar plexus
- Diaphragm
- Liver/gallbladder.

Haemorrhoids

Brief description

Haemorrhoids are caused by prolonged constipation, a diet low in fibre, not drinking enough water and lack of exercise. The main symptoms are painful bowel movements sometimes accompanied by blood in the stools, itching and inflammation of the anus.

Areas to treat

- Anus
- Large and small intestines
- Spine (especially lumbar area)
- Solar plexus
- Adrenals
- Diaphragm.

Hay fever

Brief description

Hay fever is a seasonal allergic condition which is due primarily to pollens. Hand reflexology has successfully treated many resistant cases.

Areas to treat

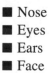

- Nose
- Eyes
- Ears
- Face

- Adrenals
- Sinuses
- Lungs
- Pituitary gland
- Lymphatics
- Large and small intestines
- Kidneys
- Neck and throat.

Headaches

Brief description

Headaches have a variety of causes. They can be caused by stress, a misalignment of the cervical vertebrae, by the sensory organs (the eyes, ears and teeth), sinusitis, hormone imbalances, allergies, digestive disorders, toxicity and tiredness.

Areas to treat

- Solar plexus
- Adrenals
- Spine – especially the cervical area
- Eyes
- Ears
- Teeth
- Head and brain
- Sinuses
- Pituitary gland
- Large and small intestines
- Liver
- All lymph glands
- Kidneys.

Heart problems

Brief description

Heart problems include angina pectoris, arrhythmia (irregular heartbeat), tachycardia (heartbeat too fast), bradycardia (heartbeat too slow), weakened heart and high blood pressure. Reflexology treatment aims to reduce stress and improve the circulation. It is important to give up smoking, take regular, gentle physical exercise and to eat a healthy diet avoiding salt, sugar, saturated fats and junk food.

Areas to treat

- Heart
- Solar plexus
- Adrenals
- Diaphragm
- Lungs
- Kidneys
- Spine
- Large and small intestines
- Liver/gallbladder.

Indigestion/heartburn

Brief description

A burning sensation behind the breastbone, which may spread up the oesophagus to the back of the mouth, is the main symptom. Heartburn may be induced by stress and tension, eating too much food and/or drink or by eating too quickly and not chewing foods properly.

Areas to treat

- Stomach/pancreas/duodenum
- Liver/gallbladder
- Adrenal glands
- Solar plexus

- Diaphragm
- Chest
- Large and small intestines.

Infertility

Brief description

Infertility, both male and female, is a very common problem. Causes include disorders or impaired function of the ovaries, fallopian tubes, uterus or a low sperm count. Stress can also decrease the chances of pregnancy. For best results both partners should be treated with hand reflexology.

Areas to treat

- Pituitary gland
- Ovaries/testes
- Uterus/prostate
- Fallopian tubes/Vas deferens
- Adrenals
- Solar plexus
- Lumbar spine
- Thyroid.

Insomia

Brief description

The majority of us suffer from periods when we find it difficult to sleep, particularly when we are under a great deal of stress. For some people it can become a major problem. Sleep-inducing drugs should only be used in the short term due to their highly addictive properties. We tend to need much less sleep as we get older and sleep requirements are variable. The worry of not getting a deep and restful sleep can prevent us from going to sleep!

Areas to treat
- Solar plexus
- Diaphragm
- Head and brain
- Lungs
- Pituitary
- Pineal
- Adrenals.

Irritable bowel syndrome

Brief description

This condition is characterized by abdominal cramping and a combination of constipation and diarrhoea. It is becoming more and more prevalent. The main cause is stress but certain foods, such as wheat and dairy foods, may be a trigger.

Areas to treat
- Large and small intestines
- Solar plexus
- Adrenals
- Stomach/pancreas/duodenum
- Liver/gallbladder
- Spine.

Liver/gallbladder problems

Brief description

These may be caused or exacerbated by alcohol, overindulging or eating the wrong foods, medications and stress. Pain is experienced particularly on the right hand side of the abdomen.

Areas to treat
- Liver
- Gallbladder
- Stomach/pancreas/duodenum

- Large and small intestines
- Spine
- Adrenals
- Solar plexus.

Male impotence

Brief description

Impotence is the inability to achieve and/or maintain an erection. A temporary state of impotence can happen to any man. Causes include physical exhaustion, nervous tension, lack of confidence and conflicts between partners.

Areas to treat

- Testes
- Vas deferens
- Prostate
- Solar plexus
- Adrenals
- Lumbar spine
- Diaphragm
- Pituitary gland
- Bladder
- Kidneys.

Menopause

Brief description

The menopause usually occurs between the ages of 45 and 55. Some women may abruptly cease menstruating, whereas for most it is a gradual process whereby an erratic cycle is experienced for years. Symptoms include hot flushes, night sweats, irregular scanty periods or heavy bleeding, irritability, depression, insomnia, memory loss, weight gain, changes in libido and vaginal dryness.

Areas to treat:

- Pituitary gland
- Ovaries
- Uterus
- Fallopian tubes
- Mammary glands
- Solar plexus
- Adrenals
- Spine
- Heart
- Lymphatics
- Thyroid/parathyroids
- Head and brain
- Kidneys.

Menstrual/ovarian disorders

Brief description

The disorders I am grouping together in this category include amenorrhoea (absence of periods), dysmenorrhoea (painful periods), endometriosis, menorrhagia (profuse bleeding), ovarian cysts, problems with the fallopian tubes and disorders of the uterus.

Areas to treat

- Ovaries
- Uterus
- Fallopian tubes
- Pituitary gland
- Lumbar spine
- Solar plexus
- Adrenals.

Migraine

Brief description

A migraine headache is frequently one-sided, excruciatingly painful and may be accompanied by sickness. Prior to an attack, dizziness and blurring of vision is very common. The tendency to suffer from migraine runs in families and may be triggered by certain foods such as cheese, chocolate and red wine. Stress is also a major factor as is lack of sleep, tiredness and irregular meals.

Areas to treat

- Head and brain
- Spine with emphasis on the neck
- Eyes
- Liver/gallbladder
- Adrenals
- Solar plexus
- Diaphragm
- Pituitary gland
- Large and small intestines
- Lymphatics
- Kidneys.

PMT

Brief description

A wide range of symptoms have been associated with PMT such as anxiety, irritability and mood swings, breast tenderness, abdominal bloating, dizziness, aggression, fluid retention, headaches, cravings for sweet things, skin problems, poor concentration and weight gain.

Areas to treat

- Pituitary gland
- Ovaries
- Uterus

■ Fallopian tubes
■ Adrenals
■ Diaphragm
■ Solar plexus
■ Head and brain
■ Pancreas
■ Spine
■ Large and small intestines
■ Lymphatics
■ Liver/gallbladder
■ Thyroid/parathyroids.

Prostate problems

Brief description

The two most common complaints are prostatitis (inflammation of the prostate) and prostatic hypertrophy (enlargement of the prostate). As men age many of them will experience enlargement of the prostate gland. Prostate symptoms include a frequent urge to urinate, pain on urination and incomplete bladder evacuation. Men should ensure that they are not suffering from carcinoma of the prostate.

Areas to treat

■ Prostate
■ Testes
■ Vas deferens
■ Adrenals
■ Solar plexus
■ Lumbar spine
■ Bladder
■ Kidneys
■ Pituitary gland
■ Pelvic lymphatics.

Sinusitis

Brief description

Sinusitis is caused by swelling of the mucous membranes that line the sinuses. It causes facial pain, particularly above and below the eyes, and may be accompanied by fever and tiredness. Toothache is another common symptom.

Areas to treat

- Sinuses
- Face
- Spine (especially cervical)
- Adrenals
- Ears
- Throat
- Eustachian tube
- Eyes
- Lungs
- Diaphragm
- Solar plexus
- Upper lymphatics
- Head and brain
- Pituitary gland
- Intestines.

Skin problems (eczema/psoriasis)

Brief description

Skin disorders include acne (already outlined), eczema and psoriasis. A common form of eczema is neurodermatitis (atopic eczema), which is an allergic condition. It may be triggered by allergens (dust mites, foods, cosmetics, medications, animal fur and pollutants), stress or by changes of season.

Psoriasis is triggered by stress and tension or environmental influences. Cell renewal can take place at ten times the normal rate resulting in scaly patches on the skin which may bleed. They occur mostly on the elbows, knees, palms of the hands and soles of the feet.

Areas to treat
- Pituitary gland
- Adrenals
- Solar plexus
- Lymphatics
- Kidneys
- Lungs
- Intestines.

Tonsillitis

Brief description

The tonsils, which are made up of lymphatic tissue, swell up in response to intruding pathogens. The symptoms are fever, pain, difficulty when swallowing and swollen lymph nodes in the neck.

Areas to treat
- Throat
- Ears
- Upper lymphatics
- Neck
- Solar plexus
- Diaphragm
- Lungs
- Adrenals.

FURTHER READING

The author, Denise Whichello Brown, is an international authority on complementary therapies. If you have enjoyed this book why not read her other books in this series:

Teach Yourself Aromatherapy – ISBN: 0 340 802707

Teach Yourself Massage – ISBN: 0 340 648112

These books, published by Hodder & Stoughton, are available through most literary outlets. If they are sold out, the bookstore can obtain a copy for you.

Useful Addresses

Beaumont College of Natural Medicine
MWB Business Exchange, Hinton Road, Bournemouth BH1 2EF
Tel: +44 (0)1202 708887 Fax: +44 (0)1202 708720
http://www.beaumontcollege.co.uk
Information on training courses under the direction of Denise Brown

Denise Brown Essential Oils
MWB Business Exchange, Hinton Road, Bournemouth BH1 2EF
Tel: +44 (0)1202 708887 Fax: +44 (0)1202 708720
http://www.denisebrown.co.uk
A wide selection of high quality pure unadulterated essential oils, base oils, creams and lotions, relaxation music, reflexology wall charts, etc. is available from Denise Brown Essential Oils (International Mail Order)

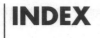

INDEX

CHARTS

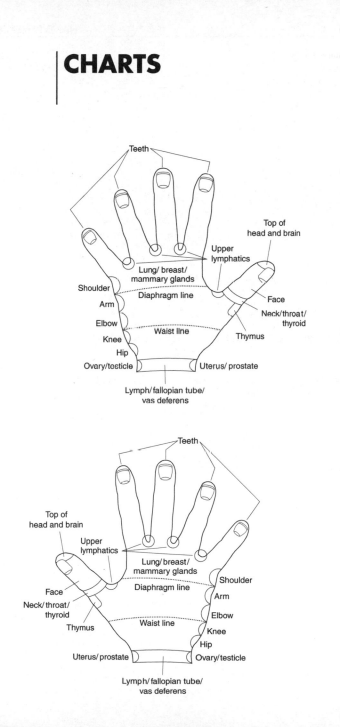

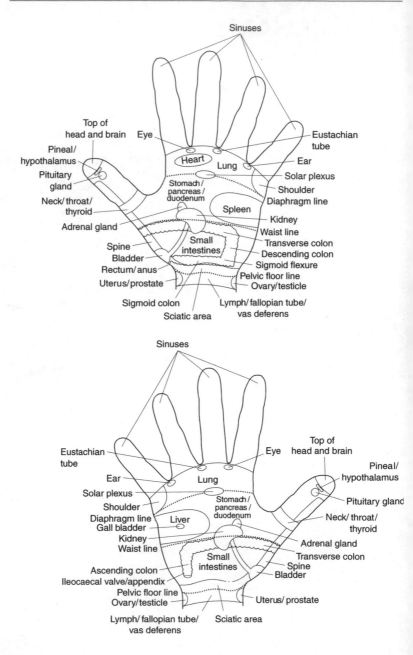